Facelift

Editors

JAMES E. ZINS
ALI H. CHARAFEDDINE

CLINICS IN PLASTIC SURGERY

www.plasticsurgery.theclinics.com

October 2019 • Volume 46 • Number 4

ELSEVIER

1600 John F. Kennedy Boulevard • Suite 1800 • Philadelphia, Pennsylvania, 19103-2899

http://www.theclinics.com

CLINICS IN PLASTIC SURGERY Volume 46, Number 4
October 2019 ISSN 0094-1298, ISBN-13: 978-0-323-69746-0

Editor: Jessica McCool
Developmental Editor: Laura Fisher

Clinics in Plastic Surgery (ISSN 0094-1298) is published quarterly by Elsevier Inc., 360 Park Avenue South, New York, NY 10010-1710. Months of issue are January, April, July, and October. Business and Editorial Offices: 1600 John F. Kennedy Blvd., Suite 1800, Philadelphia, PA 19103-2899. Periodicals postage paid at New York, NY and additional mailing offices. Subscription prices are $543.00 per year for US individuals, $940.00 per year for US institutions, $100.00 per year for US students and residents, $607.00 per year for Canadian individuals, $1119.00 per year for Canadian institutions, $649.00 per year for international individuals, $1119.00 per year for international institutions, and $305.00 per year for Canadian and international students/residents. To receive student/resident rate, orders must be accompanied by name of affiliated institution, date of term, and the *signature* of program/residency coordinator on institution letterhead. Orders will be billed at individual rate until proof of status is received. Foreign air speed delivery is included in all *Clinics* subscription prices. All prices are subject to change without notice. **POSTMASTER:** Send address changes to *Clinics in Plastic Surgery*, Elsevier Health Sciences Division, Subscription Customer Service, 3251 Riverport Lane, Maryland Heights, MO 63043. **Customer Service: 1-800-654-2452 (US and Canada). From outside of the United States and Canada, call 314-447-8871. Fax: 314-447-8029. E-mail: JournalsCustomerService-usa@elsevier.com (for print support); JournalsOnlineSupport-usa@elsevier.com (for online support).**

Reprints. For copies of 100 or more of articles in this publication, please contact the Commercial Reprints Department, Elsevier Inc., 360 Park Avenue South, New York, New York 10010-1710. Tel.: +1-212-633-3874; Fax: +1-212-633-3820; E-mail: reprints@elsevier.com.

Clinics in Plastic Surgery is covered in *Current Contents, EMBASE/Excerpta Medica, Science Citation Index, MEDLINE/PubMed (Index Medicus), ASCA, and ISI/BIOMED.*

Contributors

EDITORS

JAMES E. ZINS, MD, FACS
Chairman, Department of Plastic
Surgery, Cleveland Clinic, Cleveland, Ohio,
USA

ALI H. CHARAFEDDINE, MD
Plastic Surgeon, Center for Plastic and
Reconstructive Surgery, Adjunct Faculty,
Department of Plastic Surgery, University of
Michigan, Ann Arbor, Michigan, USA

AUTHORS

MATTEO ANGELINI, MD
Surgeon, Private Practice, Rome, Italy

RICHARD J. BEIL, MD, FACS
Plastic Surgeon, Center for Plastic and
Reconstructive Surgery, Adjunct Faculty,
University of Michigan, Ann Arbor, Michigan,
USA

PATRICK J. BUCHANAN, MD
Division of Plastic and Reconstructive Surgery,
Department of Surgery, University of Florida
Health, University of Florida College of
Medicine, Gainesville, Florida, USA

ALI H. CHARAFEDDINE, MD
Plastic Surgeon, Center for Plastic and
Reconstructive Surgery, Adjunct Faculty,
Department of Plastic Surgery, University of
Michigan, Ann Arbor, Michigan, USA

OBAID CHAUDHRY, MD
Aesthetic Plastic Surgery Fellow, Department
of Plastic Surgery, Manhattan Eye, Ear, and
Throat Hospital, New York, New York, USA

MUSTAFA CHOPAN, MD
Division of Plastic and Reconstructive Surgery,
Department of Surgery, University of Florida
Health, University of Florida College of
Medicine, Gainesville, Florida, USA

RAFAEL A. COUTO, MD
Chief Resident, Department of Plastic Surgery,
Cleveland Clinic Foundation, Cleveland, Ohio,
USA

EREZ DAYAN, MD
Plastic Surgeon, Dallas Plastic Surgery
Institute, Dallas, Texas, USA

RICHARD DRAKE, PhD
Director of Anatomy, Professor of Surgery,
Cleveland Clinic, Cleveland, Ohio, USA

PAUL D. DURAND, MD
Plastic Surgeon, Dallas Plastic Surgery
Institute, Dallas, Texas, USA

ZIYAD S. HAMMOUDEH, MD
Private Practice, Marina Plastic Surgery,
Marina Del Rey, California, USA

STEVEN LEVINE, MD
Attending, Department of Plastic Surgery,
Manhattan Eye, Ear, and Throat Hospital,
Private Practice at Steven Levine MD,
New York, New York, USA

BRUCE A. MAST, MD, FACS
Division of Plastic and Reconstructive
Surgery, Department of Surgery, University
of Florida Health, University of Florida
College of Medicine, Gainesville, Florida, USA

JENNIFER McBRIDE, PhD
Director of Virtual Anatomy Education,
Associate Professor of Surgery, Cleveland
Clinic, Cleveland, Ohio, USA

JEREMIE D. OLIVER, BS, BA
Medical Student, Mayo Clinic School of
Medicine, Rochester, Minnesota, USA

MARIO PELLE-CERAVOLO, MD
Professor, University of Padua, Padua, Italy;
Private Practice, Rome, Italy

ROD J. ROHRICH, MD
Plastic Surgeon, Dallas Plastic Surgery
Institute, Dallas, Texas, USA

KATHERINE B. SANTOSA, MD, MS
House Officer, Section of Plastic Surgery,
Department of Surgery, University of
Michigan, Ann Arbor, Michigan,
USA

W. GRANT STEVENS, MD
Private Practice, Marina Plastic Surgery,
Marina Del Rey, California, USA

CHRISTOPHER C. SUREK, DO
Assistant Professor of Anatomy, Kansas City
University, Clinical Assistant Professor of
Plastic Surgery, University of Kansas Medical
Center, Kansas City, Kansas, USA; Adjunct
Faculty, Department of Plastic Surgery,
Cleveland Clinic, Cleveland, Ohio, USA; Private
Practice, Surek Plastic Surgery, Overland Park,
Kansas, USA

GINA THOMPSON, BA
National Education Manager, Pierre Fabre
USA, Parsippany, New Jersey, USA

JAMES E. ZINS, MD, FACS
Chairman, Department of Plastic Surgery,
Cleveland Clinic, Cleveland, Ohio, USA

Contents

Facelift: History and Anatomy

Ali H. Charafeddine, Richard Drake, Jennifer McBride, and James E. Zins

In this article, we review the history of the facelift operation and how it evolved from skin excision only to the modern superficial musculoaponeurotic system operation. We describe the critical surgical anatomy of the facial layers, retaining ligaments of the face, facial spaces, the 3-dimensional complex course of the facial nerve branches, and the pertinent anatomy of the neck. This article is supplemented by fresh cadaver anatomic dissections.

The Lift-and-Fill Facelift: Superficial Musculoaponeurotic System Manipulation with Fat Compartment Augmentation

Rod J. Rohrich, Paul D. Durand, and Erez Dayan

The focus of modern face-lifting has shifted from isolated superficial musculoaponeurotic system (SMAS) manipulation to providing necessary volume restoration and overall facial shaping. Volume deflation is a major component of facial aging but cannot be corrected solely by rhytidectomy. This article presents a detailed overview of facial fat compartment anatomy and examines its role in facial rejuvenation. A good understanding of facial fat compartment anatomy cannot be overemphasized. In combination with methodical preoperative visual analysis, this allows surgeons to target the specific areas that have undergone deflation with fat grafting before selective SMAS manipulation.

Lateral SMASectomy

Obaid Chaudhry and Steven Levine

 Video content accompanies this article at http://www.plasticsurgery.theclinics.com.

The lateral superficial musculoaponeurotic system–ectomy (SMASectomy) is a safe, versatile, and easily reproducible technique in facelift surgery. The ability to resect a portion of the superficial musculoaponeurotic system (SMAS) over the junction of the mobile and fixed SMAS produces a powerful lift with similar aesthetic results to a traditional SMAS flap, but without the additional risks of nerve injury. The ability to alter the vector of motion of the underlying SMAS makes the technique adaptable to a variety of facial characteristics. The lateral SMASectomy is a viable and powerful method that has stood the test of time.

The Extended Superficial Musculoaponeurotic System

Ali H. Charafeddine and James E. Zins

The extended superficial musculoaponeurotic system (SMAS) facelift targets the 2 cardinal signs of facial aging: (1) descent of the malar fat resulting in deepening of the nasolabial folds as well as accentuation of the palpebral malar groove and tear trough deformity; (2) formation of jowls, which also obscure the definition of

skin than traction applied to the lateral platysma borders. The advantages of Lateral skin–platysma displacement are limited neck undermining, absence of submental scar, shorter operating time, faster patient recovery, satisfactory results, and an easier approach to submandibular gland reduction.

Facial volumization with filler and/or fat has become an integral part of global facial rejuvenation and provides a finishing touch to harmonize the face after surgical re-positioning of soft tissue. However, facial injection is not devoid of complications that can lead to suboptimal outcomes. This article journeys through the facial anatomy for the injector emphasizing the superficial musculoaponeurotic system as a centralized depth gauge facilitating navigation into deep and superficial injection targets. Based on this principle, the fat compartments, ligaments, potential spaces, and neurovascular structures are categorized into planes to assist the injector in performing safe and accurate volume correction.

This article discusses the various nonsurgical treatments that can be performed in combination with facelift surgery to provide patients with a more complete facial rejuvenation. Nonsurgical adjuncts focus on facial volume enhancement, skin resur-facing, intense pulsed light for pigmentary changes, neuromodulators, and skin care in addition to the surgical techniques used to combat facial aging. Several options exist for skin resurfacing, including dermabrasion, chemical peels, and lasers; the advantages and limitations of each are discussed. Photographs demonstrating the effectiveness of nonsurgical treatments to facelift patients are displayed as examples of their powerful adjunctive effect.

In this article, the authors set out to lay a foundation for successful perioperative management of the facelift patient. They describe the changes of normal facial aging in an attempt to help one recognize the universal way the face is affected by aging. Having a clear understanding of these factors may help to guide the physician with procedures necessary to offer the patient for a desired outcome. Also, the authors emphasize the preoperative assessment and postoperative care necessary to ensure a successful, low-risk operation with minimal downtime and beautiful results, meeting the patient's expectations.

CLINICS IN PLASTIC SURGERY

ISSUE OF RELATED INTEREST

Facial Plastic Surgery Clinics
https://www.facialplastic.theclinics.com/
Otolaryngologic Clinics
https://www.oto.theclinics.com/

THE CLINICS ARE AVAILABLE ONLINE!
Access your subscription at:
www.theclinics.com

Preface

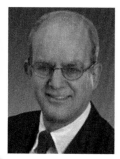 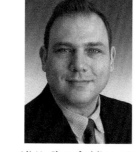

James E. Zins, MD, FACS   Ali H. Charafeddine, MD

Editors

The facelift procedure remains the cornerstone for surgical correction of the aging face. Without it, correction of facial aging cannot be complete. Mastery of the facelift operation, or more precisely delivering a consistent result, is clearly the surgeon's goal. However, the wide variety of techniques employed and the subjective and short-term nature of many of the results often depicted can leave the surgeon questioning which procedure is best for which patient.

This issue of *Clinics in Plastic Surgery* provides the practicing plastic surgeon with a detailed description of a number of the most common facelift techniques used, clear descriptions of some of the most recently described procedures, as well as the rationale for why each might work and for whom.

The issue begins with a description of the facelift anatomy emphasizing the importance of understanding the 3-dimensional nature of the area and details of the facelift danger zones where facial nerve injury is most likely. As described in the text, understanding the anatomy, superficial to deep, is critical even for those procedures that do not violate the superficial musculoaponeurotic system (SMAS).

What follows is a series of articles discussing a variety of techniques from supra-SMAS procedures, including the lateral SMASectomy and MACs lift, to the more complex sub-SMAS procedures, including the extended SMAS, and composite lift. The importance of fat grafting in facelift surgery and anatomic details regarding ideal fat graft placement are also outlined. In addition, more recently published procedures that are gaining increasing popularity, such as the lateral skin platysma displacement procedure, are described. Topics less frequently published but deserving of our attention, such as facelift after massive weight loss, and less-invasive techniques, such as the isolated or submental only approach to the neck, are addressed.

It is hoped that this issue provides the plastic surgeon with a practical framework reinforcing his/her understanding of the topic and serves as a resource for exploring areas that are as of yet untraveled.

James E. Zins, MD, FACS
Department of Plastic Surgery
Cleveland Clinic
9500 Euclid Avenue, A60
Cleveland, OH 44195, USA

Ali H. Charafeddine, MD
Center for Plastic and Reconstructive Surgery
5333 McAuley Drive, Suite 5001
Ypsilanti, MI 48197, USA

E-mail addresses:
zinsj@ccf.org (J.E. Zins)
ali_sharafeddine@hotmail.com
(A.H. Charafeddine)

Clin Plastic Surg 46 (2019) ix
https://doi.org/10.1016/j.cps.2019.07.001
0094-1298/19/© 2019 Published by Elsevier Inc.

Facelift: History and Anatomy

Ali H. Charafeddine, MD[a], Richard Drake, PhD[b], Jennifer McBride, PhD[b], James E. Zins, MD[c],*

KEYWORDS

- Facelift • SMAS • Facial nerve • Retaining ligaments

KEY POINTS

- The facelift operation significantly evolved in the past 50 years. This is mainly due to the better understanding of the complex 3-dimensional anatomy of the face. An understanding of the facial anatomy is critical for any surgeon planning a facelift.
- The description of the SMAS (superficial musculoaponeurotic system) by Mitz and Peyronie was a keystone in moving the facelift operation to the next level.
- The SMAS, galea aponeurotica, frontalis muscle, superficial temporal fascia, and platysma are all considered to be in the same plane of dissection.
- The facial nerve branches are always 1 layer deeper to the SMAS. They remain covered by the deep fascia until they exit to supply their target muscle.
- Releasing the retaining ligaments is an essential step in achieving a powerful facelift result. Understanding the anatomy of the retaining ligaments, especially as they relate to the facial nerve is key.

The fear of Surgery is the fear of Anatomy
—Ian Taylor.

INTRODUCTION

Despite the introduction of numerous nonsurgical techniques, facelift surgery remains the cornerstone of facial rejuvenation, the most powerful and durable method for correction of the facial aging process. This operation significantly evolved in the past 50 years. superficial musculoaponeurotic system (SMAS) manipulation, using either superficial plication techniques or SMAS elevation and reanchoring, is thought to be critical to success. Hence, an in-depth knowledge of the 3-dimensional anatomy of the facial layers will minimize misadventures. Controversies exist regarding the best approach to the neck during facelift surgery, with one school of thought favoring the anterior approach and the other a posterior approach.

HISTORY

Skoog[1] initiated the era of modern facelift surgery by raising a cervicofacial flap deep to the platysma in the neck and the superficial fascia in the face. Further understanding of the anatomy of the SMAS,[2] retaining ligaments,[3] and the danger zones[4] contributed to the evolution of the facelift operation. Hamra[5] and Barton[6,7] modified Skoog's[1] initial operation and likewise used a composite skin and SMAS flap in their deep plane and composite facelifts.

Owsley,[8,9] Connell,[10,11] Aston,[12] and Stuzin and colleagues[13] separated the skin from the SMAS in a bilamellar approach, to maximize vector control, despite the loss of enhanced blood supply provided by the Hamra[5] approach and the risk of potentially tearing the SMAS flap. Baker[14] and Tonnard and colleagues[15] later described the short scar and minimal access cranial suspension facelift techniques, respectively.

Disclosures: The authors have nothing to disclose.
[a] Center for Plastic & Reconstructive Surgery, P.C., 5333 McAuley Drive, Suite R5001, Ypsilanti, MI 48197, USA; [b] Cleveland Clinic, Mail Code: NA24 9500 Euclid Avenue, Cleveland, OH 44195, USA; [c] Department of Plastic Surgery, Cleveland Clinic, 9500 Euclid Avenue, A60, Cleveland, OH 44195, USA
* Corresponding author.
E-mail address: Zinsj@ccf.org

Clin Plastic Surg 46 (2019) 505–513
https://doi.org/10.1016/j.cps.2019.05.001
0094-1298/19/© 2019 Elsevier Inc. All rights reserved.

The introduction of endoscopy[16] and limited incision foreheadplasty[17] allowed forehead rejuvenation and browlift surgery to be added to the facelift operation with smaller incisions and minimal scar problems. Direct outcome comparison of these techniques to the other approaches are, however, lacking.

Other adjuncts to facelift surgery have enhanced the surgical result. This includes lipofilling, a technique popularized by the work of Coleman[18] and others,[19–21] skin resurfacing, facial implants, and lip-lifting techniques.

Skin resurfacing, whether mechanical (dermabrasion, microneedling), chemical, or energy based (lasers), leads to improvement in the quality of the skin.[22–24] Standard CO_2, fractional CO_2, erbium laser, and chemical peels have their advocates. Although full-face laser resurfacing at the time of facelift has been documented to be safe by several investigators, others recommend simultaneous peeling on nonundermined areas only.[25–28]

SURGICAL ANATOMY OF THE FACELIFT
Layers of the Face

Similar to the scalp, the face is also designed in layers. The 5 layers of the scalp, and their correspondent layers in the face are skin (layer 1), subcutaneous tissue (layer 2), galea aponeurotica (layer 3, SMAS), loose areolar tissue (layer 4, retaining ligaments and spaces), and periosteum (layer 5, deep fascia).[29] The loose areolar tissue in the scalp allows the gliding of the more superficial layers onto the deeper fixed layers (periosteum or deep temporal fascia).

The SMAS invests the muscles of facial expression and thus is necessarily a mobile structure that needs to glide on the deeper fascia. The SMAS is intimately adherent to the deep fascia in the nonmobile areas of the face, as well as in areas of ligamentous attachment or areas of fusion of the superficial and deep fascia. Although areas of dense attachments have traditionally been described as retaining ligaments (zygomatic, masseteric, mandibular), Pessa has more recently suggested that these areas represent fusion zones between the superficial and deep fascia.[29,30,31]

The deep fascia is a cranial extension of the deep cervical fascia in the neck, and corresponds to the periosteum cephalad, and the deep temporal fascia in the temple area. The proximal facial nerve branches lie deep to this fascia as they exit the parotid, making it an important landmark in facelift surgery. Of note, the plane under the deep fascia in the anterior face also contains the parotid duct and the buccal fat pad.

The Superficial Musculoaponeurotic System

The SMAS (layer 3) is a well-defined structure over the lateral face; in this area it is nonmobile and fixed to the parotid gland. The SMAS thins out as it extends medially into the cheek area and lower face. In the lower face, it tends to be more muscular, as it is in fact the cranial continuation of the platysma[2] (**Fig. 1**). The challenge in the 2-layered dissection of Marten and Stuzin is to avoid tearing of the distal SMAS during elevation.[30,32]

According to Stuzin and colleagues,[30] the SMAS invests the superficial mimetic muscles. It continues as the superficial temporal fascia in the temple area and is analog to the galea in the scalp. The SMAS is part of the superficial fascia that forms a continuous sheath throughout the head and neck area.[30]

Retaining Ligaments and Septa

The concentric layers of the face are supported in position by a series of retaining ligaments, or areas of fusion between superficial and deep fascia, that run from the deeper (fixed) structures to the dermis. The origin of the retaining ligaments can be from bone, and hence are called osteocutaneous ligaments (zygomatic and mandibular cutaneous ligaments are examples), or from confluences of the superficial and deep fascia, like the masseteric cutaneous ligaments[30] (**Fig. 2**).

The retaining ligaments or areas of fusion run in close proximity to the facial nerve branches, thus an understanding of their anatomy is critical in delivering a safe procedure.

The main zygomatic and upper masseteric retaining ligaments are located at a mean distance

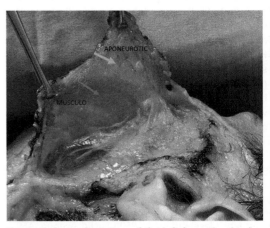

Fig. 1. Cadaver dissection of the left face. The skin has been raised and resected. The SMAS layer is raised. The SMAS is muscular (*blue arrow*) in the lower face and aponeurotic (*green arrow*) further cephalad.

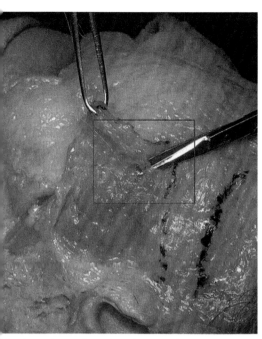

Fig. 2. Cadaver dissection showing the zygomatic retaining ligament at the inferior border of the zygomatic arch.

of 44.91 ± 9.72 mm and 46.35 ± 8.34 mm from the tragus.[4] The mandibular osteocutaneous ligament (MOCL) is the counterpart of the zygomatic retaining ligament in the lower face area. Our cadaver dissections found the MOCL to be at 56.2 ± 3.1 mm from the gonial angle along the mandibular border and 9.3 ± 1.6 mm superior to it.[33]

The platysma-mandibular ligament (PML) was described by Feldman and others,[3,33–35] and according to our cadaver dissections, is found at the anterior inferior border of the mandible.[33] The distal marginal mandibular nerve lies just superior and medial to it as it innervates the depressor anguli oris.

As mentioned earlier, the masseteric cutaneous ligaments are described as planes of fusion between the SMAS and the masseteric fascia.

Septa are defined as longitudinal lines of attachment of superficial tissue to bone or deep fascia. The superior temporal septum represents the fusion of the deep temporal fascia to the periosteum at the cranial border of the temporalis muscle. The superior temporal septum terminates at the lateral corner of the orbital rim, an area termed the temporal ligamentous adhesion.[36] The inferior temporal septum can be found extending from the superior lateral corner of the orbital rim to the external auditory canal and more importantly, the frontal branch of the facial nerve and sentinel

vein are found caudal and parallel to it. This anatomy is essential for the surgeon performing a brow lift operation[36,37] (**Fig. 3**).

The orbicularis retaining ligament (ORL), also known as the orbitomalar ligament, is a circumferential structure around the orbit that functions as an anchor of the orbicularis muscle and its overlying tissue to bone[38] (**Fig. 4**). Varying degrees of release of the ORL is critical in procedures designed to blend the lid-cheek junction as well as to access the midface through the lower eyelid incision.[11] Detailed anatomy concerning the lower eyelid rejuvenation as well as forehead rejuvenation are beyond the scope of this article.

Facial Nerve

As they exit the parotid gland, facial nerve branches lie deep to the parotid-masseteric fascia. They stay deep to this fascia and they exit into a sub-SMAS cleavage plane to innervate the undersurface of their target muscles, except 3 muscles: levator anguli oris, buccinator, and mentalis, which are innervated on their outer surface. Facial nerve branches pass through this cleavage plane distal to the retaining ligaments. Therefore, until the ligaments are encountered, nerve branches are relatively deep and out of harm's way. The frontal and marginal mandibular branches have fewer interconnections with the other branches of the facial nerve and hence pose a clinical problem if injured. Although injury

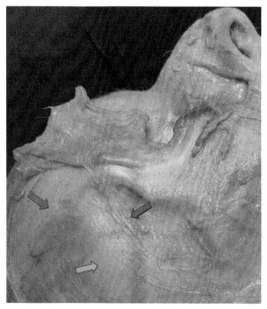

Fig. 3. Dissection of the right face. Blue arrow: Superior Temporal line. Green arrow: inferior temporal line. Red Arrow: Frontal branch of the facial nerve.

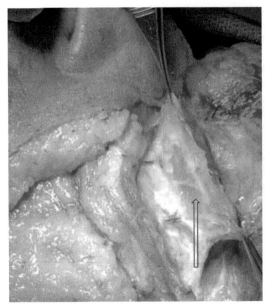

Fig. 4. Dissection of the left face. Arrow pointing at the ORL.

to the zygomatic and buccal branches can affect the patient's smile, these 2 branches have multiple interconnections making this clinically adverse outcome unlikely.[4,30]

The frontal branch anatomy as it relates to the facelift operation has been extensively studied. The original article by Pitanguy and Ramos[37] describes 4 variations in the branching pattern of the nerve. The investigators note that the direction of the "temporofrontal" branch was constant along a line projected on the skin from a point 0.5 cm below the tragus to a point 1.5 cm above the lateral "extremity of the eyebrow" (**Fig. 5**).[37]

Alghoul and colleagues[4] studied the sub-SMAS danger zone and detailed a safe passageway between the main zygomatic retaining ligament and the upper masseteric cutaneous ligament.[4] The upper zygomatic branch of the facial nerve was found consistently to be located deep to the upper third of the zygomatic major muscle and in the sub-SMAS dissection plane. The inferior zygomatic branch passes inferior to the upper masseteric ligament or at times penetrates its inferior margin. The masseteric ligaments act as sentinels to the zygomatic branches, hence the term "sub-SMAS danger zone."[4] This particular anatomy is extremely useful not only when raising the SMAS, but also when engaging maneuvers that address elevation of the malar fat pad.

The marginal mandibular nerve (MMN) has been well studied, especially as it relates to the facial artery.[39] It has on average 2.1 branches and exits the parotid gland within 1 to 2 cm of the gonial angle (**Fig. 6**). After exiting the parotid gland, the nerve crosses the facial vessels at 23.1 mm from the gonial angle along the mandibular lower border and 3.1 mm superior to it, remaining deep to the parotid-masseteric fascia. Distal to the facial vessels, the MMN is invariably found to be cranial to the lower border of the mandible, whereas before

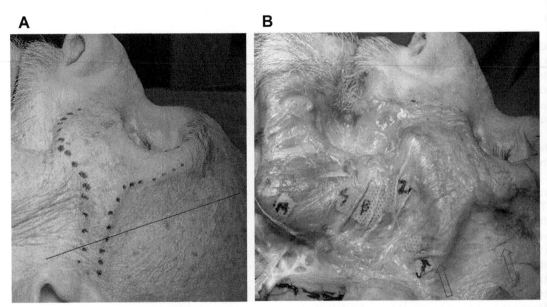

Fig. 5. (A) The Pitanguy line describes the course of the frontal branch: 0.5 cm inferior to the tragus to 1.5 cm superior to the eyebrow. (B) Left side facial nerve dissection with arrows pointing to the frontal (T) branch. B, buccal branch; M, MMN; S, stenson duct; T, temporal (frontal) branch; Z, zygomatic branch.

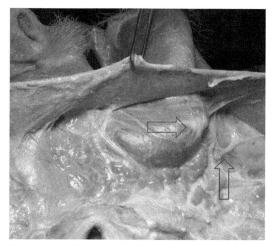

Fig. 6. Dissection of right face. Blue arrow points to the MMN. Red arrow points to the cervical branch.

it crosses the facial vessels, it is located cranial to the mandibular border 80% of the time.[33] Further distally, the MMN supplies the depressors of the lower lip.

The cervical branch supplies the platysma muscle, which is also a depressor of the corner of the mouth. An injury to the cervical branch can be differentiated from an MMN injury by asking the patient to pucker/evert his or her lower lip. If lower lip eversion is possible, this suggests that the marginal mandibular nerve is intact because the MMN innervates the mentalis (see Fig. 6). The cervical branch exits the parotid gland within 1.5 cm of the gonial angle, is under the deep investing fascia only briefly, and changes to the sub-platysmal plane. It branches into multiple rami 1.75 cm, and the most caudal branch lies 4.5 cm caudal to the lower mandibular border.[40,41]

Spaces

The complex 3-dimensional design of the SMAS and other related structures is in part responsible for the intricate nature of facial expression. This complexity accommodates, as described by Mendelson, the delicate balance "between the simultaneous needs for mobility and stability".[42] Stability is provided by the retaining ligaments of the face, responsible for binding the soft tissues of the face to either bone or deep fascia. As the facial nerve branches pass from deep to superficial, they stay in proximity with these ligaments, providing areas of stability and protection. In-between the retaining ligaments are spaces that facilitate mobility. They represent gliding planes that facilitate independent movements of the perioral and periorbital soft tissues.[43]

The prezygomatic space (PZS) is a glide plane space located over the body of the zygoma. It is triangular and bounded superiorly by the ORL and inferiorly by the zygomatic retaining ligaments. The roof of the PZS is formed by the orbicularis muscle (orbital part) and the floor is consistent with a layer of periperiosteal fat. Also, located in the floor of this space are the origins of the zygomatic major and minor muscles. There are no facial nerve branches inside this space[42] (Fig. 7).[17]

The preseptal space is located cranial to the prezygomatic space. The 2 spaces are separated by the ORL (see Fig. 7). This space provides a bloodless access to the lower eyelid.

The premaxillary space (PMS) is another bloodless gliding rectangular space overlying the maxilla. The floor of the PMS is formed by the levator labii superioris. The roof of the PMS is formed by the orbicularis oculi (orbital part) and the cheek SMAS. The upper boundary of the PMS is the ORL, whereas the lower boundary is formed by the maxillary ligaments (upper most part of the nasolabial fold at the level of the alar base).[16]

ANATOMY OF THE NECK

The neck represents an important component of the facial aging process. Therefore, neck correction is critical to a successful facelift operation. The following structures require evaluation in every planned neck rejuvenation procedure: (1) fat compartments, (2) platysma, (3) retaining ligaments, (4) digastric muscle, (5) submandibular glands, and (6) great auricular nerve (Fig. 8).

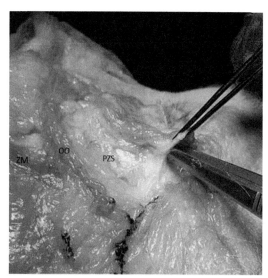

Fig. 7. Dissection in the left side of the face. The prezygomatic space is exposed through its roof (OO muscle split). Notice the surgeon entering the preseptal space with a pair of forceps.

Fat Compartments

There are 3 fat compartments in the neck: (1) superficial (supraplatysmal, which is between the skin and the platysma muscle), (2) intermediate (subplatysmal: between the platysma and the anterior digastric muscles as well as the interval between the platysma muscles), and (3) deep (deep to the digastric and submandibular glands).[44] Larsen and colleagues and Gassman and colleagues[34] showed that the superficial/supraplatysmal fat is the most abundant fat in the neck.[44] This fat is dense in nature medially and becomes less compact in the lateral aspects. The intermediate compartment contains the next greatest amount of fat. This fat is dense and fibrotic, as well as rich with blood supply and lymph nodes.[45,46] Finally, a minimal amount of fat is found in the deep compartment, and it has no clinical relevance from a neck rejuvenation standpoint.[44]

Platysma Muscles

The platysma muscles are thin sheets that originate from the clavicles and extend cranially into the SMAS (see **Fig. 1**).[2] The platysma muscles have 3 anatomic variations: type I (75%), both muscles decussate for 1 to 2 cm inferior to the symphysis menti; type II (15%), both muscles decussate from the symphysis menti all the way to the thyroid cartilage; and type III (10%), the

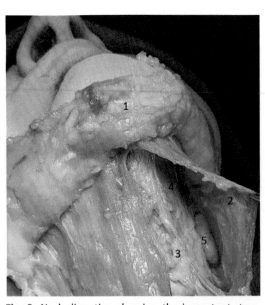

Fig. 8. Neck dissection showing the important structures to be assessed in modern neck rejuvenation surgery: 1, superficial fat (lifted up); 2, platysma; 3, subplatysmal fat; 4, digastric muscle; 5, left submandibular gland.

muscles do not meet at any point in their course.[35] Platysma laxity develops with age and tends to be most troublesome in thin necks and in patients following massive weight loss. Platysma tightening in this patient group is essential for adequate neck correction. Recurrent platysmal banding is a frequent adverse sequelae in this patient group.

Retaining Ligaments and Filaments

Joel Feldman[3] provides one of the best descriptions of the retaining ligaments and filaments of the neck. According to Feldman,[3] there are 6 ligaments in the neck: mandibular, submental, mastoid-cutaneous, platysma-auricular/ear lobe, lateral sternomastoid-cutaneous, and PMLs. There are 3 filaments: medial platysma-cutaneous, medial sternomastoid, and skin crease-platysma. These ligaments and filaments hold the neck skin in place. In addition to these ligaments and filaments, there are 3 structures that attach the platysma to the deeper structures: hyoid ligament, paramedian platysma ligament, and submandibular ligament.[35] The PML has been studied extensively, and Feldman[3] describes this ligament's course as inferior-lateral to the MOCL.[35] Rohrich more recently described the mandibular septum in a location similar to the PML.[21] We believe that these 2 structures are the same.[33,34] In our cadaver studies, the PML was found consistently at the anterior border of the masseter muscle (45.6 mm from the gonial angle along the border of the mandible).[33] Located at the anterior inferior border of the mandible, it heralds the location of the distal MMN that lies immediately superior to it.[33]

Furnas[47] described the platysma-auricular ligament as a condensation of fascia that extends from the posterior edge of the platysma to the dermis of the ear region. Feldman describes 2 different ligaments holding the ear lobe downward: the platysma-auricular and the earlobe ligaments.[3] These attachments serve as a landmark to the location of the great auricular nerve, as well as the posterior edge of the platysma. In fact, some branches of this nerve can be found on the surface of this ligament or interwoven within its fibers.[3]

The Digastric Muscles

When prominent, the anterior bellies of the digastric muscles can be partially or completely resected to help with the neck contour. This can lead to deepening of the cervicomental angle secondary to the unopposed pull of the hyoid retractors.[48]

The digastric muscles are essential in understanding the anatomy of the neck, as they are part of the submental as well as the submandibular triangles.[45] The hyoid forms the inferior border of the submental triangle, whereas the anterior bellies of the digastrics form its superolateral edges. The symphysis menti forms the apex of the submental triangle, and the mylohyoid muscle is its floor.[49]

The submandibular triangle is formed by both the anterior and posterior bellies of the digastric and the lower edge of the mandible (superior margin). This triangle hosts the following important structures: submandibular glands, facial vessels, lingual nerve, and MMN. Thus, a thorough understanding of this anatomy is key when planning a neck rejuvenation procedure, especially those involving submandibular gland resection.[50]

Submandibular Glands

The submandibular glands, when prominent, can contribute to bulges or irregularities of the neck/jawline and hence affect the aesthetic outcome. This is especially true after the skin is tightened and aggressive neck defatting is performed in thin necks. The gland is invested by the deep cervical fascia, and is composed of superficial and deep lobes that lie superficial and deep to the mylohyoid muscle respectively.[51] The superficial lobe is the larger of the 2 and is the one partially resected during surgery.[45,49]

Singer and Sullivan[52] studied the anatomy of the submandibular gland and its relation to the important nearby neurovascular structures in 15 fresh fixed cadavers. The MMN was located external to the gland capsule and 3.7 cm cephalad to the inferior margin of the gland. The lingual nerve crosses the submandibular gland duct anteriorly and is located under the mandibular border. The vascular anatomy is variable, with on average 1.5 vessels entering the superficial lobe medially, 1 intermediate vessel also entering medially to supply both the superficial and deep lobes, and 1 central vessel entering centrally from the deep lobe to the superficial lobe.[51]

Mendelson and Tutino[53] described their experience in submandibular gland resection in 112 patients. They report major complications in 1.8% of patients requiring reoperation for significant hematomas (1 potentially fatal). Minor complications were reported at 10.8% (managed nonoperatively). The most frequent complications were submandibular sialocele (4.5%) and marginal mandibular neurapraxia (4.5%), and all were resolved by 3 months. In their series, no patient reported a permanent dry mouth.[52]

Resection of the submandibular gland for aesthetic reasons remains an area of debate.

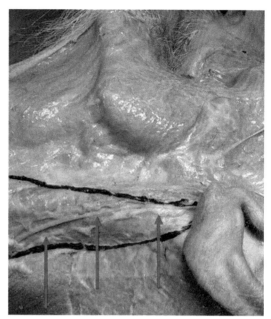

Fig. 9. Dissection of the left side of the face. Shown is the great auricular nerve (*red arrows*) within the boundaries of the Ozturk triangle.

Those who are against it believe it places many important structures at risk. Others believe that it is critical to a successful neck rejuvenation.[54,55]

Great Auricular Nerve

The great auricular nerve is reportedly the most frequently injured nerve during facelift surgery. The hyperesthesia that results from its injury usually resolves. However, problems from nerve entrapment or neuroma formation can be debilitating. McKinney and Katrana[56] located the nerve 6.5 cm inferior to the external acoustic meatus at the midbelly of the sternocleidomastoid muscle.

Ozturk and colleagues[57] described a failsafe method to avoid injury to the great auricular nerve during rhytidectomy (**Fig. 9**). This method relies on defining the danger zone of the great auricular nerve early in the facelift operation. This zone is defined by a vertical line perpendicular to Frankfurt horizontal plane, bisecting the lobule of the ear, and another arm extending posteriorly at 30°.[54]

SUMMARY

The signs of aging that affect the face, such as deepening of the nasolabial folds, formation of marionette lines and jowls, and sagging of the midface area, are all related to the 3-dimensional anatomy that we discussed in this article. It is also important to understand that this anatomy is highly variable, based on all the cadaveric studies that we now have available. A meticulous understanding of this anatomy is crucial for the plastic surgeon planning a facelift operation.

REFERENCES

1. Skoog T. New methods and refinements. Plastic surgery. 1st edition. Stokholm (Sweden): Almgrist and wicksell International; 1974. p. 300–30.
2. Mitz V. Peyronie. M. The superficial musculoaponeurotic system (SMAS) in the parotid and cheek area. Plast Reconstr Surg 1976;58(1):80–8.
3. Feldman JJ. Surgical anatomy of the neck. Necklift. 1st edition. Stuttgart (Germany): Thieme; 2006. p. 106–13.
4. Alghoul M, Bitik O, McBride J, et al. Relationship of the zygomatic facial nerve to the retaining ligaments of the face: the sub-SMAS danger zone. Plast Reconstr Surg 2013;131(2):245e–52e.
5. Hamra ST. The deep plane rhytidectomy. Plast Reconstr Surg 1990;86(1):53–61 [discussion: 62–3].
6. Barton FE. The SMAS and the nasolabial fold. Plast Reconstr Surg 1992;89:1054–9.
7. Barton FE. The "high SMAS" face lift technique. Aesthet Surg J 2002;22:481–6.
8. Owsley JQ. Platysma-fascial rhytidectomy: a preliminary report. Plast Reconstr Surg 1977;60: 843–50.
9. Owsley JQ. SMAS-platysma face lift. Plast Reconstr Surg 1983;71:573–6.
10. Connell BF. Eyebrow, face, and neck lifts for males. Clin Plast Surg 1978;5:15–28.
11. Connell BF, Marten TJ. The trifurcated SMAS flap: three-part segmentation of the conventional flap for improved results in the midface, cheek, and neck. Aesthetic Plast Surg 1995;19:415–20.
12. Aston SJ. Platysma-SMAS cervicofacial rhytidoplasty. Clin Plast Surg 1983;10:507–20.
13. Stuzin JM, Baker TJ, Gordon HL, et al. Extended SMAS dissection as an approach to midface rejuvenation. Clin Plast Surg 1995;22:295–311.
14. Baker DC. Lateral SMASectomy. Plast Reconstr Surg 1997;100:509–13.
15. Tonnard P, Verpaele A, Monstrey S, et al. Minimal access cranial suspension lift: a modified S-lift. Plast Reconstr Surg 2002;109:2074–86.
16. Vasconez LO, Core GB, Gamboa-Bobadilla M, et al. Endoscopic techniques in coronal brow lifting. Plast Reconstr Surg 1994;94:788–93.
17. Knize DM. Limited incision foreheadplasty. Plast Reconstr Surg 1999;103:271–90.
18. Coleman SR. Long-term survival of fat transplants: controlled demonstrations. Aesthetic Plast Surg 1995;19:421–5.
19. Guerrerosantos J. Simultaneous rhytidoplasty and lipoinjection: a comprehensive aesthetic surgical strategy. Plast Reconstr Surg 1998;102:191–9.
20. Tonnard P, Verpaele A, Peeters G, et al. Nanofat grafting: basic research and clinical applications. Plast Reconstr Surg 2013;132:1017–26.
21. Rohrich RJ, Ghavami A, Constantine FC, et al. Lift-and-fill face lift. Plast Reconstr Surg 2014;133(6): 756e–67e.
22. Baker TJ. Chemical face peeling and rhytidectomy. A combined approach for facial rejuvenation. Plast Reconstr Surg Transplant Bull 1962;29:199–207.
23. Baker TJ, Gordon HL. Chemical face peeling: an adjunct to surgical facelifting. South Med J 1963; 56:412–4.
24. Stuzin JM, Baker TJ, Gordon HL. Treatment of photoaging. Facial chemical peeling (phenol and trichloroacetic acid) and dermabrasion. Clin Plast Surg 1993;20(1):9–25.
25. Ozturk CN, Huettner F, Ozturk C, et al. Outcomes assessment of combination face lift and perioral phenol-croton oil peel. Plast Reconstr Surg 2013; 132(5):743e–53e.
26. Orra S, Waltzman JT, Mlynek K, et al. Periorbital PhenolCroton oil chemical peel in conjunction with blepharoplasty: an evolving technique for periorbital facial rejuvenation. Plast Reconstr Surg 2015;136: 99–100.
27. Carruthers JD, Carruthers JA. Treatment of glabellar frown lines with *C. botulinum*-A exotoxin. J Dermatol Surg Oncol 1992;18:17–21.
28. Duranti F, Salti G, Bovani B, et al. Injectable hyaluronic acid gel for soft tissue augmentation. A clinical and histological study. Dermatol Surg 1998;24: 1317–25.
29. Shaw RB, Kahn DM. Aging of the midface bony elements: a three dimensional computed tomographic study. Plast Reconstr Surg 2007;119(2): 675–81.
30. Stuzin JM, Baker TJ, Gordon HL. The relationship of the superficial and deep facial fascias: relevance to rhytidectomy and aging. Plast Reconstr Surg 1992; 89(3):441–9 [discussion: 450–1].
31. Pessa JE. SMAS Fusion Zones Determine the Subfascial and Subcutaneous Anatomy of the Human Face: Fascial Spaces, Fat Compartments, and Models of Facial Aging. Aesthet Surg J 2016;36(5): 515–26.
32. Marten TJ1. High SMAS facelift: combined single flap lifting of the jawline, cheek, and midface. Clin Plast Surg 2008;35(4):569–603.
33. Huettner F, Rueda S, Ozturk CN, et al. The relationship of the marginal mandibular nerve to the mandibular osseocutaneous ligament and lesser ligaments of the lower face. Aesthet Surg J 2015;35(2): 111–20.
34. Gassman AA, Pezeshk R, Scheuer JF 3rd, et al. Anatomical and clinical implications of the deep and superficial fat compartments of the neck. Plast Reconstr Surg 2017;140(3):405e–14e.

35. de Castro CC. The anatomy of the platysma muscle. Plast Reconstr Surg 1980;66(5):680–3.

36. Moss CJ, Mendelson BC, Taylor GI. Surgical anatomy of the ligamentous attachments in the temple and periorbital regions. Plast Reconstr Surg 2000; 105(4):1475–90 [discussion: 1491–8].

37. Pitanguy I, Ramos S. The frontal branch of the facial nerve: the importance of its variations in face lifting. Plast Reconstr Surg 1966;(38):352–6.

38. Muzaffar AR, Mendelson BC, Adams WP Jr. Surgical anatomy of the ligamentous attachments of the lower lid and lateral canthus. Plast Reconstr Surg 2002;110(3):873–84 [discussion: 897–911].

39. Dingman RO, Grabb WC. Surgical anatomy of the mandibular ramus of the facial nerve based on the dissection of 100 facial halves. Plast Reconstr Surg Transplant Bull 1962;29:266–72.

40. Salinas NL, Jackson O, Dunham B, et al. Anatomical dissection and modified Sihler stain of the lower branches of the facial nerve. Plast Reconstr Surg 2009;124:1905–15.

41. Chowdhry S, Yoder EM, Cooperman RD, et al. Locating the cervical motor branch of the facial nerve: anatomy and clinical application. Plast Reconstr Surg 2010;126:875–9.

42. Mendelson BC, Muzaffar AR, Adams WP. Surgical anatomy of the midcheek and malar mounds. Plast Reconstr Surg 2002;110:885–96.

43. Wong C-H, Mendelson B. Facial soft-tissue spaces and retaining ligaments of the midcheek: defining the premaxillary space. Plast Reconstr Surg 2013; 132(1):49–56.

44. Larson JD, Tierney WS, Ozturk CN, et al. Defining the fat compartments in the neck: a cadaver study. Aesthet Surg J 2014;34(4):499–506.

45. Reece EM, Pessa JE, Rohrich RJ. The mandibular septum: anatomical observations of the jowls in aging—implications for facial rejuvenation. Plast Reconstr Surg 2008;121(4):1414–20.

46. Ramirez OM. Multidimensional evaluation and surgical approaches to neck rejuvenation. Clin Plast Surg 2014;41(1):99–107.

47. Furnas DW. The retaining ligaments of the cheek. Plast Reconstr Surg 1989;83(1):11–6.

48. Guyuron B. Problem neck, hyoid bone, and submental myotomy. Plast Reconstr Surg 1992;90(5): 830–7 [discussion: 838–40].

49. Kohan EJ, Wirth GA. Anatomy of the neck. Clin Plast Surg 2014;41(1):1–6.

50. Zins JE, Waltzman J, Couto RA. Neck rejuvenation. In: Rubin P, Neligan P, editors. Plastic surgery volume 2: aesthetic surgery. 4th edition. Oxford (United Kingdom): Elsevier; 2017. p. 375–89.

51. Last RJ. The head and neck. Anatomy regional and applied. 7th edition. New York: Churchill Livingstone; 1984. p. 17–8.

52. Singer DP, Sullivan PK. Submandibular gland I: an anatomic evaluation and surgical approach to submandibular gland resection for facial rejuvenation. Plast Reconstr Surg 2003;112(4):1150–4 [discussion: 1155–6].

53. Mendelson BC, Tutino R. Submandibular gland reduction in aesthetic surgery of the neck: review of 112 consecutive cases. Plast Reconstr Surg 2015;136(3):463–71.

54. Marten T, Elyassnia D. Short scar neck lift: neck lift using a submental incision only [review]. Clin Plast Surg 2018;45(4):585–600.

55. de Pina DP, Quinta WC. Aesthetic resection of the submandibular salivary gland. Plast Reconstr Surg 1991;88(5):779–87 [discussion: 788].

56. McKinney P, Katrana DJ. Prevention of injury to the great auricular nerve during rhytidectomy. Plast Reconstr Surg 1980;66(5):675–9.

57. Ozturk CN, Ozturk C, Huettner F, et al. A failsafe method to avoid injury to the great auricular nerve. Aesthet Surg J 2014;34(1):16–21.

The Lift-and-Fill Facelift
Superficial Musculoaponeurotic System Manipulation with Fat Compartment Augmentation

Rod J. Rohrich, MD, Paul D. Durand, MD*, Erez Dayan, MD

KEYWORDS

• Facelift • Rhytidectomy • Fat compartments • SMAS plication • SMAS stacking

KEY POINTS

- Current facelift techniques have shifted from the single focus of superficial musculoaponeurotic system (SMAS) alteration to volume restoration and facial recontouring.
- The deep malar (medial) compartment and nasolabial fold are always fat grafted first, whereas the high lateral (superficial) compartment is augmented last.
- SMAS stacking is typically indicated for facial sides that are narrower and require more fullness.
- SMASectomy is indicated for wider and fuller faces.

INTRODUCTION

Current facelift techniques have shifted from the single focus of superficial musculoaponeurotic system (SMAS) alteration to volume restoration and facial recontouring. Although tissue mobilization and elevation remain a mainstay in facial rejuvenation, restoring volume is what allows a smooth contour and overall facial shaping. A combination of such techniques, appropriately tailored for each face, is what allows the natural and enduring result that patients request.[1,2]

The lift-and-fill facelift combines an individualized alteration of the SMAS with precise volume augmentation. It is now understood that deflation is a major component of the complex facial aging phenomenon and cannot be corrected by rhytidectomy alone. Anatomic studies have provided a topographic map of the superficial and deep facial fat compartments. Surgeons can now accurately and precisely augment areas that have undergone such deflation while the SMAS and its involved structures are selectively repositioned.[1–5]

Fill of Deep and Superficial Fat Compartments

Several studies have suggested that facial subcutaneous fat is highly compartmentalized.[3,4,6,7] In a youthful face the transition between subcutaneous compartments is smooth, whereas in aging individuals there are abrupt contour changes between these regions. An in-depth understanding of these compartments has proved invaluable for the successful correction of facial aging. Through cadaveric studies, Rohrich and Pessa[3] first revealed the superficial facial compartments[3,7] (**Fig. 1**).

Indications for specific fat compartment augmentation are based on preoperative analysis of the topographic deflation. Accurate preoperative planning of selective fat compartment grafting is the first step in the lift-and-fill facelift. The deep volumetric foundation influences the extent and type of SMAS and skin manipulation. SMAS stacking is performed

Disclosures: Dr R.J. Rohrich receives instrument royalties from Eriem Surgical, Inc., and book royalties from Thieme Medical Publishing. No funding was received for this article. Dr P.D. Durand and Dr E. Dayan have no financial interests to declare in relation to the content of this article.
Dallas Plastic Surgery Institute, 9101 North Central Expressway, Suite 600, Dallas, TX 75231, USA
* Corresponding author.
E-mail address: pdurand85@gmail.com

Clin Plastic Surg 46 (2019) 515–522
https://doi.org/10.1016/j.cps.2019.06.001

Superficial Facial Fat Pads

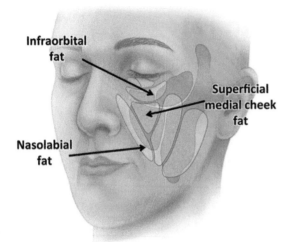

Deep Facial Fat Pads

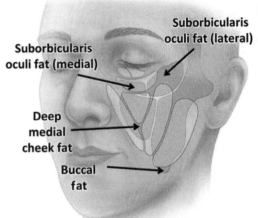

Fig. 1. Anatomy of both superficial (*left*) and deep (*right*) facial fat compartments. (*From* Pessa JE, Rohrich RJ. Facial Topography: Clinical Anatomy of the Face. St. Louis: Quality Medical Publishing; 2012; with permission.)

superficial to the augmented deeper malar compartments. In the setting of a fuller and/or wider facial side, where SMASectomy would be preferred, fat transfer volumes may be less indicated in the high lateral malar compartment to enhance the desired contour.[1,2,6]

An intimate relationship exists between the fat compartments and retaining ligaments of the face. Retaining ligaments are often noted to arise from areas of fascial coalescence at the junction between fat compartments. The superficial fat compartments of the face are divided by septal barriers arising from the SMAS. In the midface, these include part of the nasolabial fat and the lateral, middle, and medial cheek fat. These observations clinically correlate with those areas of fixation that are encountered when dissecting a hemiface from lateral to medial. Zones of fixation correspond with transition areas between compartments and typically have some vascular component.[3,7]

The nasolabial compartment is bordered superiorly by the orbicularis retaining ligament; the nasolabial fat compartment is distinct and can be noted medial to the deeper fat of the suborbicularis fat compartment. The lower border of the zygomaticus major muscle is adherent to this compartment. In the cheek area, there are 3 distinct fat compartments: the medial, middle, and lateral-temporal cheek fat. The medial cheek fat is found lateral to the nasolabial fold and is bordered superiorly by the orbicularis retaining ligament and the lateral orbital compartment. Inferior to the medial cheek compartment lies the jowl fat. The middle cheek

fat is found anterior and superficial to the parotid gland. In its superior portion, it is partially adherent to the zygomaticus major. Where these 3 superficial compartments meet, a confluence of septa occurs and is where the zygomatic ligament is commonly described. The zone where the medial fat compartment abuts that of the middle cheek compartment corresponds with the parotidomasseteric ligaments.[3,7]

The lateral-temporal cheek compartment is the most lateral compartment of cheek fat. It lies just superficial to the parotid gland, bridging the temporal fat to the cervical subcutaneous fat. The first transition zone encountered during a facelift when advancing medially from the preauricular incision corresponds with a true septum located anterior to the lateral-temporal fat compartment.[3,7]

Although the superficial fat compartments can be manipulated by SMAS suspension to a certain extent, the deep fat of the midface is primarily altered using volume. Deep fat compartments include the deep malar (medial) compartment, middle malar, nasolabial fold, and superior cheek. The deep malar (medial) compartment lies beneath the orbicularis oculi muscle and is bounded laterally by the capsule of the buccal fat pad and the zygomaticus major muscle. The pyriform ligament surrounding the nasal base forms the medial boundary and the orbital retaining ligament its superior limit. The deep medical cheek fat was found to be supplied mainly by the infraorbital artery.[1,3,7]

Separate from nasolabial fat is the jowl fat compartment, the most inferior fat on the face. In this area, fat is adherent to the depressor anguli oris muscle, which also makes for its medial-most boundary. Superiorly, jowl fat is bordered by naso-labial fat and medial fat, and inferiorly by the mem-branous fusion of the platysma muscle.[3]

The deep malar (medial) compartment and naso-labial fold are always fat grafted first, whereas the high lateral (superficial) compartment is augmented last. The deep malar compartment should be seen as the workhorse compartment in effective volume restoration[1,3,6] (**Fig. 2**). Considering that, in this area, fat lobule size is smaller and deflates at an accelerated rate, it should always be augmented first.[8] The injection of fat deep and medial to the zygomaticus major muscle significantly improves midface projection, resulting in a more youthful cheek.[1,3,6]

After adequate augmentation of the deep com-partments, the surgeon can proceed to fill the more superficial areas of the face. The nasolabial fold is filled first and then the high lateral cheek can be addressed. Although this serves to accen-tuate malar highlights in women, it should be cir-cumvented in men to avoid a feminizing effect.[9] Filling the middle and lateral superficial malar com-partments can aid in blending the lower cheek junc-tion and nasojugal crease.[1,3,6] In addition, perioral compartments can help augment the inferior naso-labial region and soften perioral rhytides.[10]

Fat Harvesting and Injection Technique

Various fat harvesting and preparation techniques have been discussed in the literature.[11,12] The inner thigh and abdomen have been shown to contain the highest concentration of stromal vascular cells and are of small cell size.[13] In our practice, manual low-pressure lipoaspiration of the inner thigh is accomplished using a blunt 3-mm cannula with multiple small holes. The lipoaspirate should fill

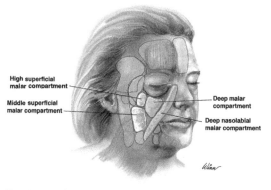

High superficial malar compartment
Middle superficial malar compartment
Deep malar compartment
Deep nasolabial malar compartment

Fig. 2. Key fat compartments to be filled as part of the lift-and-fill facelift. (*From* Rohrich RJ, Ghavami A, Constantine FC, et al. Lift-and-fill face lift: inte-grating the fat compartments. Plast Reconstr Surg 2014;133(6):761e; with permission.)

approximately half of a 10-mL syringe and is placed in a centrifuge for no longer than 1 minute (2250 rev-olutions/min) at low pressure to remove cellular debris. The isolated middle fat should be trans-ferred to a 1-mL syringe and promptly injected. Approximately 10 to 12 mL of yellow fat is distrib-uted into the 2 deep central facial fat compart-ments. Another 10 to 20 mL is then injected in between the nasolabial compartment and lateral compartments depending on the augmentation desired. In men, the high superficial malar and mid-dle superficial malar compartments are avoided to avoid feminization of the face.[1,4,6]

It is recommended for fat transfer to take place at the beginning of the procedure, not only to decrease the chance of fat environmental contam-ination but also to allow for accurate tailoring of the SMAS over the augmented fat compartments. A 16-gauge needle is used to introduce a blunt-tipped Coleman cannula for deep compartment injection. For injection of the superficial compart-ments, a 21-gauge needle directly attached to the syringe can be used, which allows more pre-cise injection and minimizes vascular trauma when injecting thicker subdermal tissue.[1,4,6]

Selective Skin Undermining

Before local anesthetic infiltration, incision place-ment is planned. The senior author prefers to use an intratragal incision that extends perpendicular to the preauricular incision along the infratemporal hairline anteriorly. The latter extension of the inci-sion allows proper vertical redraping of the elevated skin flap. As with any incision in the hairline, bevel-ing of the blade minimizes chances of alopecia. The inferior portion of the incision always extends around the base of the ear lobule and around the conchal cartilage. Incision placement in the poste-rior ear takes place a few millimeters above the postauricular sulcus because there is a tendency for this scar to descend as healing occurs. The inci-sion then extends superiorly along the hairline, tailoring its length to how much skin excess is being removed.[1,2,5,9]

Once placement of the incision has been marked, the superwet technique is used for infiltra-tion. This infiltration technique is defined as having a volume greater than 50 to 100 mL per hemiface. The solution is mixed preoperatively and consists of 30 mL of 0.5% lidocaine and 1.5 mL of epineph-rine 1:1000, all mixed in 300 mL of normal saline. It is injected in the subcutaneous plane where skin flap dissection is planned using a 22-gauge spinal needle on an autofill syringe. A long spinal needle inserted only along the incision line avoids trauma to the skin flap and allows uniform hydrodissection in a plane between the skin flap and SMAS. Hydro-dissection with the superwet technique has proved particularly useful in secondary facelifts. About 90 to 120 mL of fluid is infiltrated per hemi-face. The total volume injected is guided by the presence of moderate skin turgor without skin blanching. In order to maximize the vasoconstric-tive effects of the epinephrine, at least 15 minutes is allowed to pass between injection time and the start of skin elevation. The incision site is rein-jected before final closure.[2,14]

The senior author has always used a 2-layer approach that separates skin and SMAS layers. This approach allows bidirectional vector move-ment and more natural skin redraping. The level of skin undermining should be dictated by the shape and width of the patient's face. In the past, skin flap undermining usually extended medially to the nasolabial groove, which has the possibility of nasal groove effacement, oral commissure distortion, and compromising vascularity. An individualized approach serves to limit skin undermining to either the lateral canthus or just medial to the zygomaticus major muscle. In those patients with minimal skin

laxity and in faces with a wide malar width, advancing the medial SMAS laterally may not be necessary and, thus, skin undermining does not need to be extensive. In contrast, patients with narrow faces that need volume recruited cephalad toward the zygomatic arch benefit from wider undermining.[2,5]

Superficial Musculoaponeurotic System and Platysma Manipulation

Skin-based techniques, although safer and possibly quicker, do not retain the same visco-elastic properties as SMAS system approaches. Procedures that allow the SMAS to bear the load of the subcutaneous mass and overall soft-tissue tension are associated with greater longevity.[5,15] It has not been clearly determined whether there is 1 specific method of SMAS manipulation that works better than other techniques. Techniques that cen-ter on SMASectomy or SMAS plication/imbrication with adequate skin undermining obviate extended SMAS dissection and can still provide excellent outcomes.[1,2,16,17]

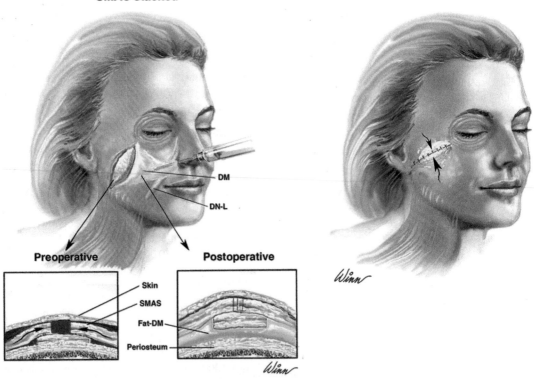

Fig. 3. In the SMAS-stacking technique, the SMAS is carefully incised, undermined proximally and distally, and then advanced toward a central axis line. When the undermined edges are brought over the remaining SMAS base, a 3-layered stacking effect results in enhanced malar projection and cheek fullness. DM, deep malar; DN-L, deep nasolabial fold. (*From* Rohrich RJ, Ghavami A, Constantine FC, et al. Lift-and-fill face lift: integrating the fat compartments. Plast Reconstr Surg 2014;133(6):761e; with permission.)

An individualized component facelift approach not only allows varying vectors of pull but also serves in better tailoring differing techniques of SMAS manipulation to each face. Preoperative evaluation of facial length and fullness dictates the orientation or angle of SMAS shaping and direction of SMAS movement. SMAS stacking is typically indicated for facial sides that are narrower and require more fullness. Such faces are in sharp contrast to those wider and fuller faces that better benefit from SMA-Sectomy. The former not only allows enhanced augmentation in the precise topographic location that is indicated but also helps bridge the contouring effect between the deep medial and lateral superficial malar compartments.[1–6,9]

In the SMAS-stacking technique, the SMAS is carefully incised, undermined proximally and distally, and then advanced toward a central axis line. When the undermined edges are brought over the remaining SMAS base, a 3-layered stacking effect results in enhanced malar projection and cheek fullness. Stacking is a more powerful augmentative maneuver than plication because an island of SMAS is preserved centrally and a bilaminar construct is created[1–6,9] (Fig. 3).

The exact location of where the SMAS is incised is important because this affects where the augmentation occurs with the stacking technique. The amount of SMAS incorporated in each individual stitch bite can also serve to tailor the extent of the augmentation. Furthermore, the underlying skeletal support affects the area that is to be augmented. Patients with strong skeletal support, such as those with a greater interzygomatic width and more prominent malar eminences, may not require as much SMAS stacking over the lateral malar region. This facial shape is likely to benefit more from a horizontally directed SMAS layering or SMASectomy that mobilizes tissue in a vertical vector[1–6,9] (Fig. 4).

The importance of a well-defined neck contour in facial rejuvenation cannot be overstated. In patients without platysmal banding, the senior author addresses the neck using a lateral platysma window. This technique was devised in order to minimize complications during neck lifting, particularly great auricular nerve injury. Incision for the platysma window is marked anterior to the lobule at 1 fingerbreadth below the angle of the mandible and 1 fingerbreadth in front of the anterior border of the sternocleidomastoid muscle. A platysma window that is 2 cm in vertical length is performed by elevating the platysma using forceps and electrocautery. When enough of a flap has been elevated to allow good traction power, the dissection stops. It is then sutured to the posterior mastoid fascia using 2 figure-of-eight 4-0 Mersilene

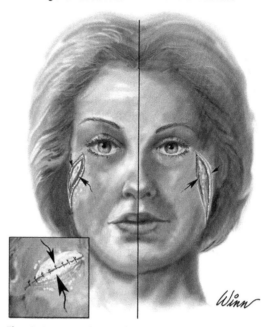

Stacked SMAS
Long and Narrow Face

SMASectomy
Short and Wide Face

Fig. 4. Preoperative evaluation of facial length and fullness dictates the orientation or angle of SMAS shaping and direction of SMAS movement. SMAS stacking is typically indicated for facial sides that are narrower and require more fullness, whereas SMASectomy is more appropriate in fuller and/or wider facial sides. (*From* Rohrich RJ, Ghavami A, Constantine FC, et al. Lift-and-fill face lift: integrating the fat compartments. Plast Reconstr Surg 2014;133(6):762e; with permission.)

sutures (Ethicon, Inc.), spanning the area where the great auricular nerve is located.[2,5,18,19]

When platysmal banding is present, an anterior platysmaplasty is performed using a submental incision. This approach allows correction of medial platysmal laxity and also resection of subplatysmal fat under direct visualization in those select cases in which this is indicated. If a medial plastymaplasty is needed, the senior author performs this after the SMAS has been fixated. This order of events allows maximal malar elevation without having an opposing pull if the midline plication is performed first. Placement of the submental incision is planned posterior to the submental crease in order to prevent excessive deepening of the crease. Skin flap elevation in this area is done just above the platysma with most of the fat remaining attached to the skin. Wide skin undermining occurs in order to communicate with the lateral skin flaps already previously dissected. Using electrocautery, the medial borders of the platysma are defined, followed by removal of excess fat in between these. Platysmaplasty is then performed using interrupted figure-of-eight sutures from inferior to superior. Inferiorly, the muscle is then transected transversely right above the thyroid cartilage, accentuating the cervicomental angle.[2,5,18,19]

Platelet-rich plasma is used by the senior author before closure of the skin incision in order to decrease postoperative bruising, swelling, and total drain output.[20] While the patient is being prepped, venous blood is drawn with a 60-mL syringe containing 6 mL of anticoagulant and centrifuged. A 10-mL dual-port sprayer syringe is used to draw up the platelet-rich plasma. It is then sprayed in between the skin flap and the underlying SMAS.[1,2,9,20] In an effort to reduce intraoperative bleeding and postoperative hematoma, the senior author now uses tranexamic acid both topically and intravenously. Its antifibrinolytic effect has been extensively studied in other surgical specialties and now is becoming more widely adopted in plastic surgery. For topical administration, tranexamic acid is diluted to a 3% concentration in order to

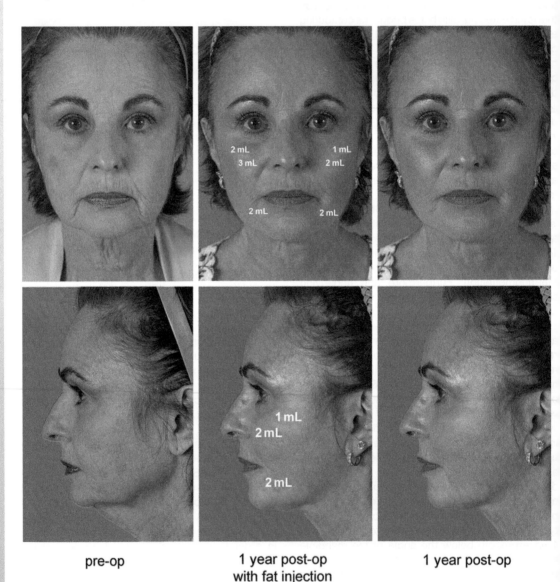

pre-op   1 year post-op with fat injection   1 year post-op

Fig. 5. A 60-year-old woman after a lift-and-fill facelift combined with individualized manipulation of the SMAS. Fat transfer volumes and their locations are labeled. SMAS stacking was performed bilaterally but in a more oblique vector on the right and with more undermining to address the shorter/wider facial side. Patient also underwent medial platysmaplasty through an anterior open approach. post-op, postoperative; pre-op, preoperative. (*From* Rohrich RJ, Ghavami A, Constantine FC, et al. Lift-and-fill face lift: integrating the fat compartments. Plast Reconstr Surg 2014;133(6):763e; with permission.)

be applied directly over the wound for 3 to 5 minutes at the end of surgery. In patients in whom the surgical site is especially bloody or in those at a higher risk of postoperative bleeding (eg, male patients), 1 g of tranexamic acid is administered intravenously during surgery.[21]

DISCUSSION

It is now understood that deflation is a major component of facial aging and, thus, cannot be corrected solely by rhytidectomy. The focus of modern face-lifting has shifted from isolated SMAS manipulation to providing necessary volume restoration and facial shaping. Precise volume augmentation should not be viewed as just an adjunct to rhytidectomy but more as a crucial component in facial rejuvenation. Patients who undergo lipofilling at the time of facelift report significantly higher satisfaction compared with those undergoing a facelift alone[1,2,22] (Fig. 5).

Once thought of as an anatomically continuous structure, the subcutaneous fat of the face has been shown to be highly compartmentalized.[3] Septal boundaries separating facial compartments are composed of a vascularized fibrous membrane carrying an identifiable perforator supplying the skin.[3,7] The most medial of the major cheek compartments, the nasolabial fat, is separated from the upper lip fat by the nasolabial septum. Within this septum run perforator vessels from the angular artery. The most lateral fat compartment is the lateral-temporal cheek fat, and this is supplied by perforators arising from the branches of the superficial temporal artery. Medial to the lateral-temporal cheek compartment is the middle cheek fat. The middle cheek septum, which forms the medial limit of this compartment, contains perforating branches from the transverse facial artery to the overlying skin. Located in between the middle cheek fat and nasolabial fat is the medial fat compartment, supplied by perforators of the facial and infraorbital arteries.[3,7]

Although the changes that occur with facial aging are not fully understood, this is most likely a multifactorial phenomenon. The idea of retaining ligament attenuation as the sole culprit of facial aging has been disproved. In his observations of midface and periorbital aging, Lambros[23] shows that the true descent of soft tissues might not be as profound once thought, showing that the lid-cheek junction does not typically descend with age.[1,3,23] A more likely cause for facial aging is the formation of separations between the already defined fat compartments. Loss of midface fullness, particularly in the malar and submalar areas, indicates the aging face and can only be corrected with precise fat augmentation. SMAS-shaping techniques, such as stacking, can further contribute to restoring volume in the malar region in the deflated midface. This combination is so powerful that the senior author routinely uses some degree of fat compartment augmentation of the deep malar, nasolabial, and oral commissures at the time of every facelift.[1–6,10]

The lift-and-fill facelift combines precise volume augmentation with individualized alteration of the SMAS. A good understanding of facial fat compartment anatomy cannot be overemphasized. In combination with a methodical preoperative, topographic visual analysis, this allows surgeons to target the specific areas that have undergone deflation with fat grafting before selective SMAS alteration. The outcome of such individualized combination of techniques results in the successful comprehensive correction of the aging face.

REFERENCES

1. Rohrich RJ, Ghavami A, Constantine FC, et al. Lift-and-fill face lift: integrating the fat compartments. Plast Reconstr Surg 2014;133(6):756e–67e.
2. Rohrich RJ, Ghavami A, Lemmon JA, et al. The individualized component face lift: developing a systematic approach to facial rejuvenation. Plast Reconstr Surg 2009;123(3):1050–63.
3. Rohrich RJ, Pessa JE. The fat compartments of the face: anatomy and clinical implications for cosmetic surgery. Plast Reconstr Surg 2007;119(7):2219–27.
4. Rohrich RJ, Pessa JE, Ristow B. The youthful cheek and the deep medial fat compartment. Plast Reconstr Surg 2008;121(6):2107–12.
5. Rohrich RJ, Narasimhan K. Long-term results in face lifting: observational results and evolution of technique. Plast Reconstr Surg 2016;138(1):97–108.
6. Pezeshk RA, Small KH, Rohrich RJ. Filling the facial compartments during a face lift. Plast Reconstr Surg 2015;136(4):704–5.
7. Schaverien MV, Pessa JE, Rohrich RJ. Vascularized membranes determine the anatomical boundaries of the subcutaneous fat compartments. Plast Reconstr Surg 2009;123(2):695–700.
8. Wan D, Amirlak B, Giessler P, et al. The differing adipocyte morphologies of deep versus superficial midfacial fat compartments: a cadaveric study. Plast Reconstr Surg 2014;133(5):615e–22e.
9. Rohrich RJ, Stuzin JM, Ramanadham S, et al. The modern male rhytidectomy: lessons learned. Plast Reconstr Surg 2017;139(2):295–307.
10. Pezeshk RA, Stark RY, Small KH, et al. Role of autologous fat transfer to the superficial fat compartments for perioral rejuvenation. Plast Reconstr Surg 2015;136(3):301e–9e.

11. Bucky LP, Percec I. The science of autologous fat grafting: views on current and future approaches to neoadipogenesis. Aesthet Surg J 2008;28(3): 313–21.

12. Hsu VM, Stransky CA, Bucky LP, et al. Fat grafting's past, present, and future: why adipose tissue is emerging as a critical link to the advancement of regenerative medicine. Aesthet Surg J 2012;32(7): 892–9.

13. Geissler PJ, Davis K, Roostaeian J, et al. Improving fat transfer viability: the role of aging, body mass index, and harvest site. Plast Reconstr Surg 2014; 134(2):227–32.

14. Costa CR, Ramanadham SR, O'reilly E, et al. The role of the superwet technique in face lift: an analysis of 1089 patients over 23 years. Plast Reconstr Surg 2015;135(6):1566–72.

15. Saulis AS, Lautenschlager EP, Mustoe TA, et al. Biomechanical and viscoelastic properties of skin, SMAS, and composite flaps as they pertain to rhytidectomy. Plast Reconstr Surg 2002;110(2):590–8.

16. Guyuron B, Rowe DJ, Weinfeld AB, et al. Factors contributing to the facial aging of identical twins. Plast Reconstr Surg 2009;123(4):1321–31.

17. Ivy EJ, Lorenc ZP, Aston SJ. Is there a difference? a prospective study comparing lateral and standard SMAS face lifts with extended SMAS and composite rhytidectomies. Plast Reconstr Surg 1996;98(7): 1135–43.

18. Narasimhan K, Stuzin JM, Rohrich RJ. Five-step neck lift: integrating anatomy with clinical practice to optimize results. Plast Reconstr Surg 2013; 132(2):339–50.

19. Pezeshk RA, Sieber DA, Rohrich RH. Neck rejuvenation through the lateral platysma window: a key component of face-lift surgery. Plast Reconstr Surg 2017;139(4):865–6.

20. Brown SA, Appelt EA, Lipschitz A, et al. Platelet gel sealant use in rhytidectomy. Plast Reconstr Surg 2006;118(4):1019–25.

21. Rohrich RJ, Cho MJ. The role of tranexamic acid in plastic surgery: review and technical considerations. Plast Reconstr Surg 2018;141(2):507–15.

22. Kappos EA, Temp M, Schaefer DJ, et al. Validating facial aesthetic surgery results with the FACE-Q. Plast Reconstr Surg 2017;139(4):839–45.

23. Lambros V. Observations on periorbital and midface aging. Plast Reconstr Surg 2007;120:1367–76.

Lateral SMASectomy

Obaid Chaudhry, MD[a],*, Steven Levine, MD[b]

KEYWORDS

- Facelift • Lateral SMASectomy • Plication • Short-scar facelift • Facelift incision • Facelift vectors
- Biplanar facelift • Necklift

KEY POINTS

- The lateral superficial musculoaponeurotic system rhytidectomy is a safe, versatile method for manipulating the underlying superficial musculoaponeurotic system (SMAS) in a facelift.
- Sub-SMAS techniques have not been proved to provide a superior aesthetic outcome and only result in higher risk of injury to deeper structures.
- Skin vector manipulation and incision placement are just as important as SMAS techniques.
- Preauricular and intratragal incisions are used based on patient characteristics
- SMAS plication is an alternative approach in secondary patients or those with underappreciated SMAS tissue.

 Video content accompanies this article at http://www.plasticsurgery.theclinics.com.

INTRODUCTION

The evolutionary change of facelift techniques has varied from skin-only procedures to more superficial musculoaponeurotic system (SMAS)–oriented techniques.[1–8] The manipulation and elevation of the SMAS was initially published in 1976 by Mitz and Peyronie,[9] and this was at the time, and for many years following, deemed the proper way to achieve superior results in facelift surgery. However, it was noted by Daniel Baker[1,2] that this deep dissection over the lateral, fixed SMAS, which overlapped the parotid gland, did not provide a significant difference in the facial form. Furthermore, Dr Baker noted that elevating the anterior SMAS did little to provide any meaningful benefit for most patients, and put them at risk for facial nerve injuries. The quality of the anterior SMAS raising a flap was noted to be thin with intermittent tears, and unable to hold any significant sutures, thus leading to early relapse.[1–8,10–12]

In 1992, the lateral SMASectomy was conceptualized and brought to fruition by Dr Baker.[1,7] A strip of SMAS is undermined and excised parallel to the nasolabial fold at the junction of the mobile and fixed SMAS. This strip of SMAS overlays the anterior aspect parotid gland, with minimal overlap in a danger zone. Following this excision, the more mobile anterior SMAS is approximated to the fixed posterior SMAS, leading to a vector that is usually perpendicular to the nasolabial fold. The key concept of identifying the junction of the mobile and fixed SMAS, and using its ability to move ptotic tissues to the immobile deep tissue, results in long lasting and excellent results. The result is an improved jawline, jowl, and cervical skin with effacement of the nasolabial fold. Later, in 2001, the short-scar facelift was developed, which was geared toward women in their 40s who did not desire a posterior incision, which at times can become unappealing with distortion, pigment changes, or widening.[1,10,11]

Disclosure: The authors have nothing to disclose.
[a] Department of Plastic Surgery, Manhattan Eye, Ear, and Throat Hospital, 210 East 64th Street, 3rd Floor, New York City, NY 10065, USA; [b] Department of Plastic Surgery, Manhattan Eye, Ear, and Throat Hospital, Private Practice at Steven Levine MD, 210 East 64th Street, 3rd Floor, New York City, NY 10065, USA
* Corresponding author.
E-mail address: obachaudhry@gmail.com
; @DrOCPlasticSurg (O.C.); @StevenLevineMD (S.L.)

LATERAL SMASECTOMY VERSUS DEEP PLANE TECHNIQUES

It is easy to be persuaded that deeper, more aggressive techniques provide a stronger, or more long-lasting, lift. However, no data exist to support this concept.[13,14] The best study examining this difference in technique fairly definitively showed, at best, a lack of superiority of the deep plane techniques, and, by some observers, an inferiority.[13] What this study reveals is that the biggest difference between plastic surgeons is not technique but aesthetic judgment. How much to pull and what vector to move is more important than technique.

With the recent push toward less invasive procedures and rapid recovery, the use of these more invasive procedures, which include SMAS flaps, composite, and deep plane approaches, may become less popular in the near future. Less scarring, bruising, bleeding, and risk, and a quicker recovery, now present a more attractive option for many patients. With a short-scar approach, the absence of a retroauricular incision and maintenance of the hairline is a strong appeal to many women, especially those who prefer their hair in ponytails or pulled back.

It is not our intention to doubt these deep plane techniques, but we question their risk/benefit ratio. The real question is whether or not these provide a significant long-term benefit, and, if so, do the risks and complications of these procedures offset the supposed added value to the overall outcome. It is our belief that differences in results are based on the techniques of individual surgeons, who may have different aesthetic ideals.

There are many advantages of the lateral SMA-Sectomy. The risk of tearing the anterior superficial fascia is decreased because there is no flap elevation. In addition, the risk to the facial nerve is diminished because the SMAS resection is mainly performed over the parotid gland. Also, because the possibility of tearing the fascia is much less than with traditional flap procedures, suture fixation is more reliable, with a lower chance of so-called cheesewiring, leading to a longer-lasting result. Although the lateral SMASectomy is one of the most reliable techniques used by the senior author, surgeons must tailor their methods to each patient. For example, an SMAS plication is likely a better option for someone who is thin skinned with little to no subcutaneous fat. The end goal should be a repeatable, effective, reliable, and safe procedure that is translatable across a wide spectrum of patients.

Skin redraping and incision planning are equally important factors that must not be overlooked for a natural, elegant result. When performing a biplanar technique, in which the skin is separated from the underlying SMAS, surgeons have the capability of using 2 different vectors for each layer of tissue. This capability can be individualized to each patient's specific aesthetic needs.

Incision placement is generally an overlooked, but important, concept for achieving an excellent result. Whether a preauricular or intratragal incision is used depends on numerous patient factors, which include gender, skin characteristics, hair quality and hairline, and natural creases. It is important to redrape without distorting the aesthetic subunits of the ear or hairline. A poorly executed incision and skin vector will be evident and mask any excellent SMAS manipulation.

PATIENT EVALUATION AND SELECTION

The lateral SMASectomy can be applied to a wide range of patients, from full-face patients to average, typical-face patients. The person who may not be first choice is a person in whom the surgeon does not want to sacrifice volume, therefore SMAS plication and/or stacking are favored, which affects the facial tissue in near-identical ways with complete preservation of SMAS as opposed to removal of volume. The lateral SMASectomy elevates the cheek, improves jowls, and helps efface the nasolabial folds. This option is almost always combined with a neck procedure, involving wide undermining, either with a lateral SMASectomy by itself or a midline platysmaplasty, or both.

OPERATIVE PROCEDURE
Anesthesia

Most facelifts are performed under monitored anesthesia care with intravenous propofol sedation. Preoperative clonidine, 0.1 to 0.2 mg, is given orally to aid in blood pressure control. A tumescent solution consisting of 0.5% lidocaine with 1:200,000 epinephrine via a 22-gauge spinal needle is infiltrated in the face and neck. This stage is done before a betadine preparation because this aids in a 10-minute time period for the vasoconstrictive effect to occur.

Incisions

When assessing incision placement, the quality and characteristics of the hairline must be considered. If the shift of the hairline is minimal, then an incision placed in the temporal hairline is desired. Redundant tissue may need to be excised just below the temporal sideburn at the level of the root of the helix if this incision pattern is performed. Although this design moves the hairline, this may be suitable if there is a small amount of movement if the hairline is naturally low.

If there is a greater amount of skin movement (as with a short-scar facelift when the lift is in a vertical vector), or if the distance between the lateral canthus and temporal hairline is greater than 5 cm, an incision a few millimeters within the temporal hairline is recommended. This option is preferable to elevating the hairline, which would be the result of an incision within the temporal hairline. When these properly planned incisions are healed, they are generally imperceptible, except in darker-skinned individuals, in whom the scar may appear hypopigmented and contrast with the natural skin tone. The incision in the temporal hair is placed parallel to the hair follicle and does not extend higher than the frontotemporal region. As shown by Camirand and Doucet,[15] the incision must be beveled toward the flap, or perpendicular to the hair follicles, so future hair growth may occur within the scar. With the anterior temporal hairline incision, a vertical lift is achievable, which is required in patients with excessive skin laxity, or those with a recessed hairline and thinning hair from previous facelift surgery (**Fig. 1**).

A preauricular versus intratragal incision depends on surgeon preference and patient factors. The senior author uses both incision types and makes a choice dependent on what suits the patient best. No single incision pattern is best for all patients. If performed in a proper manner, a preauricular incision heals without issue and is not noticeable, and most importantly preserves the tragal unit. With this technique, the incision is curved in front of the helix and continues down anterior to the tragus in a natural fold. This method prevents the coarse, thick, dark cheek skin with lanugo hairs that results from unnaturally being placed over the tragus, where skin is generally thin, hairless, and pale. Intratragal incisions can be placed in patients in whom the tragal and cheek skin are similar and the tragal cartilage is blunted and not sharp or prominent. This method results in less scar burden on the face. If this is performed, the closure over the tragus must be without tension, and the authors prefer to defat the skin flap over the tragus to the level of the dermis at this area.

With a short-scar approach, the incision usually ends at the level of the earlobe. At times, a small dog-ear may be present, but this can be removed with a small retroauricular incision after flap inset.

Skin Flap Elevation

The skin flap is undermined using sharp scissor dissection under direct visualization. This method

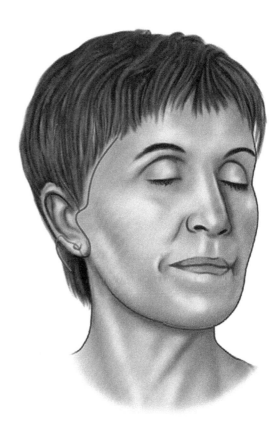

Fig. 1. Incision placement for facelift. These incisions can be in the anterior hairline, which aids in a more vertical lift, versus a temporal incision, which can shift the hairline back. An intratragal or preauricular incision is placed based on skin characteristics, prominence of a skin fold, and hair location. The extent of the postauricular incision depends on neck laxity; a short-scar approach stops at the ear lobe or continues to a minimum amount posteriorly, versus a full-scar approach into the hairline, which is more appropriate for patients with significant skin laxity.

minimizes trauma to the subdermal plexus and conserves a layer of subcutaneous fat on the skin flap. The temporal region is undermined in the subcutaneous plane as well because this allows the skin to redrape easily (hair loss is caused by tension, and not a superficial dissection).[1] The surgeon must carefully dissect in this area and avoid piercing the superficial temporal fascia that covers the frontal branch of the facial nerve. The dermal attachments between the skin and orbicularis oculi muscle are usually released up to the level of the lateral canthus.

The dissection should release the zygomatic ligaments over the zygoma but should stop a few centimeters before the nasolabial fold. In the senior author's opinion, there is little to no benefit in an extended skin dissection, and it leads to a higher risk of bleeding. The masseteric-cutaneous ligaments must be released in the cheek, and, if required, the mandibular-cutaneous ligaments.

The elevation of the flap must continue over the mandibular angle and sternocleidomastoid for 5 to 6 cm into the neck. This elevation reveals the posterior portion of the plastysma. If the patient is a candidate for a submental incision, the lateral and facial flap elevation is connected via the submental incision.

Defatting the Neck and Jowls

The use of closed suction-assisted lipoplasty is the preferred to alternative methods for sculpting the neck. The authors use a 2.4-mm Mercedes tip cannula, making sure to keep it under constant, steady movements in the subcutaneous space. A layer of subcutaneous fat is preserved on the cervical skin, and, if the jowls are suctioned, this is done in a conservative fashion.

Subplatysmal fat is seldom removed because (1) the facial nerve is in danger and lies just under the platysma muscle; and (2) patients with significant subplatysmal fat usually also have fat, round faces, so removal of the subplatysmal fat may result in an overoperated, unnatural appearance.

The lipoplasty is generally performed before elevation of the skin flaps. Care is taken to not oversuction the portion of the SMAS-platysma that will be raised over the mandible with a lateral SMASectomy. Surgeons should be conservative with liposuction at the beginning of the surgery because more can always be removed at the end.

Open Submental Incision with Medial Platysma Approximation

In many patients, closed suction-assisted liposuction and a strong lateral platysmal pull provide excellent results. However, the best results are achieved by opening the neck and directly addressing the platysma. In patients with strong active platysmal bands on animation, medial approximation of the platysma provides an additional vector to enhance the cervicomental contour (**Fig. 2**). Other techniques, including the lateral skin platysma displacement, originally described by Guerrero-Santos and colleagues[16] in 1974, and more recently Pelle-Ceravollo and colleagues,[17] use a lateral-only composite skin muscle flap approach to obtain excellent neck contour. Our preferred technique is to open the midline neck and address the platysmal bands directly. All of these techniques, as with SMAS techniques, are variations on a theme.

With a midline approach, the submental incision can be made either in the crease or just

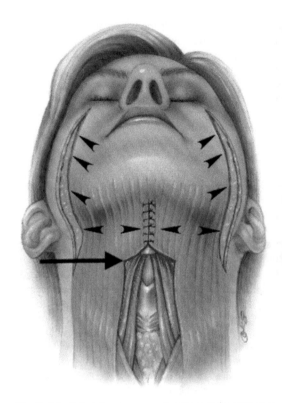

Fig. 2. Medial platysma approximation. Subcutaneous dissection through a submental incision is performed with the neck hyperextended. The dissection usually extends to the level of the thyroid cartilage and angle of the mandible. Suction-assisted lipoplasty is then performed. The medial borders of the platysma muscle are elevated for several centimeters. To break the continuity of the bands, a wedge of muscle is removed at the level of the hyoid (*black arrow*). The medial borders of the muscle are then sutured together. The vector of movement of the SMAS and platysma is represented in an oblique manner and towards the midline, respectively (*black arrowheads*). (*From* Baker DC, Levine SM. Lateral SMASectomy and facelift. In: Azzizzadeh B, Murphy M, Johnson C, et al, editors. Master techniques in facial rejuvenation. 2nd ed. Toronto: Elsevier; 2018. p. 214; with permission.)

directly anterior to it. Whether an incision is made directly in the crease, anterior, or posterior depends on surgeon preference or exposure. The senior author prefers an incision in the crease based on anecdotal data, but any location can yield excellent results. If access to the submandibular glands is necessary, then the incision should be placed posterior to the crease. If made anterior to the crease, the ligaments within the crease should be released. The dissection is performed in a subcutaneous plane with the neck hyperextended. The dissection is carried to the level of the thyroid cartilage and mandibular angle. Following this, suction-assisted lipoplasty is then performed with a large, single-hole cannula under direct visualization. Fat can be directly excised if required, but subplatysmal fat is rarely removed.

The medial borders of the platysma are identified and flaps are elevated for several centimeters, either with blunt dissection or electrocautery. In order to break the continuity of the bands and prevent possible reoccurrence, a small wedge of muscle is excised at the level of the hyoid bone, or a full transection. At times, it is necessary to excise redundant platysma. Next, the medial borders of the platysma muscle are sutured together in the middle with interrupted buried 4-0 polydioxanone (PDS; Ethicon, Inc., Somerville, NJ) sutures. An imbricating running absorbable suture may be placed over this repair to prevent any contour irregularities. The submental incision is left open until the end of the procedure to aid in final hemostasis and recontouring after communication with the facial skin flap and the lateral SMASectomy has been completed.

Lateral SMASectomy Including Platysmal Resection

The lateral SMASectomy outline is marked on a tangent from the lateral malar eminence to the angle of the mandible, which is along the anterior edge of the parotid gland (**Fig. 3**). This line of excision usually extends from the lateral aspect of the malar eminence to the tail of the parotid gland in most patients. The key landmarks are within this range. The mobile SMAS laxity is variable, and the surgeon must lift up this area with forceps to judge the amount of resection and motion that can be achieved. Depending on SMAS-platysma laxity, around 2 to 3 cm of superficial fascia is resected.

In the SMAS excision, the superficial fascia at the area of the parotid gland tail must be picked up, and the resection continued from inferior to superior in a meticulous manner. When SMAS resection is being executed, it is vital to stay superficial to the deep fascia in order to avoid removing part of the parotid parenchyma. Keep in mind that there is a varying degree of thickness of parotid gland among patients, and thus there is a variable degree of protection of the facial nerve between different patients. As long as the surgeon stays superficial to the deep fascia while performing the SMASectomy, facial nerve and parotid gland injury will be avoided. Anterior to the parotid gland, there is minimal protection of the

facial nerve and the buccal branches are not protected. The plane of dissection is similar to if an SMAS flap were to be raised (Video 1). The elevation of the lateral platysma and lateral platysmaplasty must be performed first to prepare for the lateral SMASectomy because of creation of a dog-ear. Essentially, the lateral SMASectomy can be thought of an excision of a dog-ear of SMAS (**Fig. 4**).

Removal of a strip of platysma posteriorly along the tail of the parotid gland and anterior border of the sternocleidomastoid muscle is in continuity with the lateral SMASectomy. This area of resection is safe because the facial nerves are protected.

Vectors

There are numerous vectors that aid in the improvement of the anterior neck, cervicomental angle, jowls, and nasolabial fold. The initial suture holds the lateral platysma at the mandibular angle and advances it in a posterior-superior vector to the fixed lateral SMAS with a 2-0 Maxon (United States Surgical Corp., Norwalk, CT). This key suture lifts the cervical platysma and cervical skin.

Next, the authors use interrupted 3-0 absorbable, monofilament, buried sutures to close the SMASectomy, with the fixed lateral SMAS being uniformly sutured to the mobile anterior superficial fascia. This method produces a vector that is often perpendicular to the nasolabial fold (**Fig. 5**). The final suture lifts the malar fat pad, which then fixates it to the malar fascia on the anterior cheek. If necessary, the suture line can be oversawn with a 4-0 monofilament suture and/or the area trimmed with the back of the scissors to prevent any contour irregularities. Secure fixation is vital in order to prevent postoperative dehiscence and relapse of the original facial contour (see **Fig. 4C**).

Monofilament sutures such as PDS or Maxon should be buried and sharp ends on the knot are cut in order to prevent any palpability postoperatively. Any final contouring of the SMAS or fat irregularities may be performed along the fixation line with direct excision. The sternomandibular trough fat can be excised if necessary to highlight the mandibular angles, and additional contouring may be performed with suction-assisted lipoplasty.

For improvement of the neck, a lateral platysmal flap or window is developed in the area of the inferior mandibular border. After the platysmal flap has been elevated, it is secured to the mastoid fascia with a figure-of-eight 2-0 Maxon suture to aid in

A

B

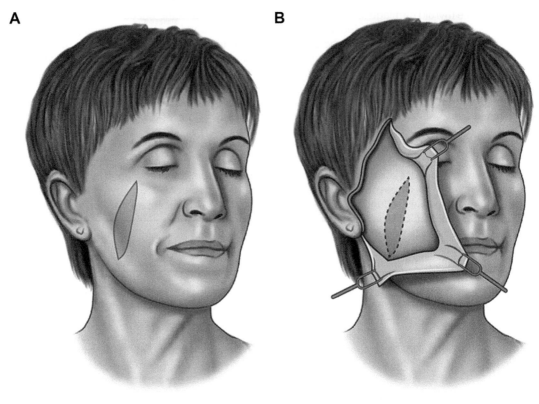

Fig. 3. (A) Proposed outline and design of the lateral SMASectomy. (B) Skin flaps elevated with the design of the lateral SMASectomy. The resection level must stay superficial to the parotid-masseteric fascia to prevent facial nerve injury. (C) An oblique vector of movement is shown, in which the more anterior, mobile SMAS is relocated to the area of the fixed SMAS.

C

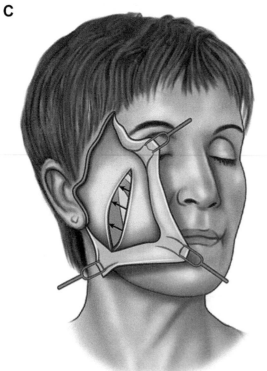

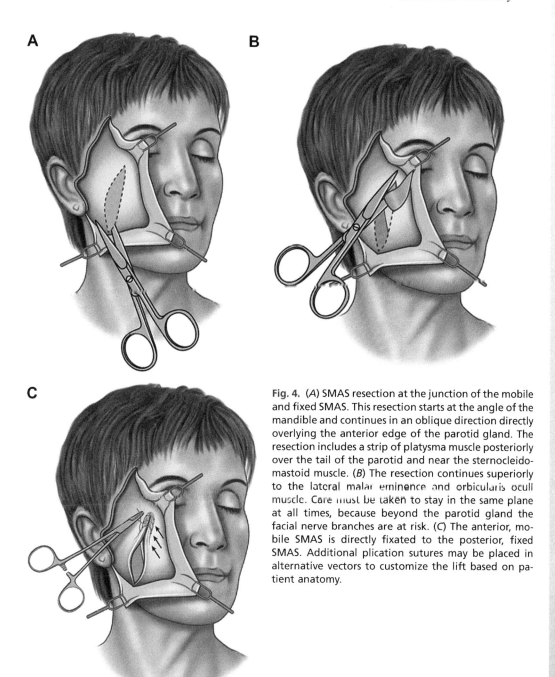

Fig. 4. (A) SMAS resection at the junction of the mobile and fixed SMAS. This resection starts at the angle of the mandible and continues in an oblique direction directly overlying the anterior edge of the parotid gland. The resection includes a strip of platysma muscle posteriorly over the tail of the parotid and near the sternocleido-mastoid muscle. (B) The resection continues superiorly to the lateral malar eminence and orbicularis oculi muscle. Care must be taken to stay in the same plane at all times, because beyond the parotid gland the facial nerve branches are at risk. (C) The anterior, mobile SMAS is directly fixated to the posterior, fixed SMAS. Additional plication sutures may be placed in alternative vectors to customize the lift based on patient anatomy.

jawline definition and improve submandibular silhouette. The platysmal flap may also be performed in conjunction with a midline platysmaplasty or in isolation, depending on individual anatomy.

Skin Closure, Temporal and Earlobe Dog-Ears

Once the SMAS and platysma have been approximated, there may be gathering of the skin at the anterior extent of the subcutaneous dissection as a result of the pull of the underlying SMAS. This

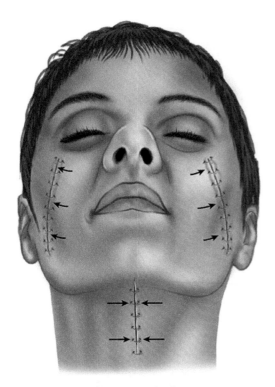

Fig. 5. Vectors of SMAS and platysma movement noted in the face and neck, respectively.

tethering may also occur in the lower eyelid secondary to elevation of the malar fat pad. An additional subcutaneous dissection must be performed in order to free and release these dimples, thus allowing the skin to redrape smoothly. A key point is to only undermine as needed to release these dimples, because creating unnecessary dead space risks more complications without added benefit.

The initial key suture rotates the facial flap in a vertical and posterior direction in order to elevate the midface, jowls, and submandibular skin. Suture fixation is performed at the level of the superior helix with a buried 3-0 PDS suture through the temporal fascia with a significant bite of dermis on the skin flap in order to prevent strain on the skin closure. Closure of the flap must be under minimal to moderate tension. Staples are used to close incisions in the hair. In order to preserve the hairline, a wedge of skin is usually removed at the level of the sideburn. If a pretrichial incision is used, this is closed with buried 5-0 Monocryl (Ethicon, Inc.) and 5-0 nylon sutures for the skin. Surgeons must spend ample time and care on closure of the skin flap to prevent dog-ear formation and acquire a fine scar. Any excess skin is cut from the facial flap so no tension is placed on the preauricular closure. The edges of the wound

should be "kissing" without any sutures in order to prevent scar widening (**Fig. 6**).

The skin flap must be trimmed at the earlobe without tension, and the skin is placed under the lobe with 4-0 PDS sutures, which takes a bite of the earlobe dermis, cheek flap dermis, and conchal perichondrium to reduce any tension. A closed suction drain is brought through a separate stab incision in the posterior ear sulcus. **Figs. 7** and **8** show preoperative and postoperative lateral SMASectomy patients.

POSTOPERATIVE CARE

The main concern postoperatively is a hematoma, especially in the first 48 hours. Thus, continuous blood pressure monitoring is required in order to prevent any systolic pressure increases and bleeding. Increased blood pressure must be treated in order to prevent postoperative hematomas.[18]

The senior authors use closed suction drains and a soft head dressing to cover the incisions and flaps. Drains are used to remove any

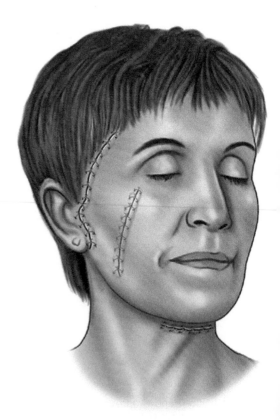

Fig. 6. SMAS, platysma, and skin closure in the lateral SMASectomy. Note that multiple sutures at different levels are needed for the midline platysma plication. Shown is 1 level of plication of the platysma.

A

B

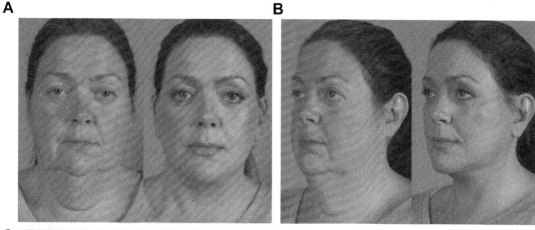

C

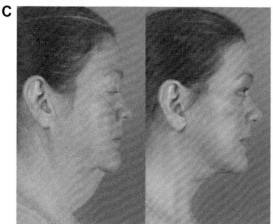

Fig. 7. Anterior (*A*), oblique (*B*), and lateral (*C*) preoperative and 1-year postoperative views of a 49-year-old female lateral SMASectomy patient. Of note, she also had a chin implant for her microgenia.

serosanguinous fluid, although they do not prevent hematoma. Drains are usually removed within 24 hours; however, they may be kept in longer depending on output. Skin sutures can be removed on postoperative day 7 to 10.

The hematoma rate for women is about 1.5%, and up to 4% in men.[2,18] These hematomas must be addressed promptly to prevent long-term negative sequelae such as skin sloughing,

A

B

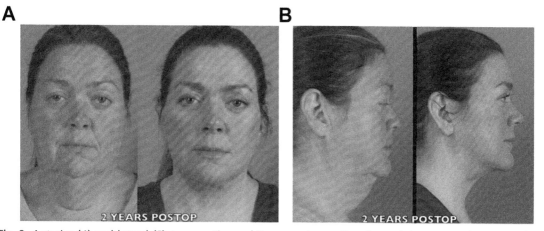

Fig. 8. Anterior (*A*) and lateral (*B*) preoperative and 2-year postoperative views of the same patient. Note the maintenance of neck contour and malar fullness.

Table 1
Complications associated with 3500 lateral SMASectomy facelifts

Complication	Incidence (%)
Hematoma (female/male)	1.5/4.0
Facial nerve weakness	0.1[a]
Earlobe scar revision	2.0
Skin slough	2.0
Retroauricular and temporal scar revisions	2.0
Infection	1.0
Minilift after 1 y	2.0

[a] All resolved within 6 months.

From Baker DC, Levine SM. Lateral SMASectomy and facelift. In: Azzizzadeh B, Murphy M, Johnson C, et al, editors. Master techniques in facial rejuvenation. 2nd ed. Toronto: Elsevier; 2018. p. 218; with permission.

necrosis, or induration, leading to a poor aesthetic outcome.

COMPLICATIONS

Common complications are listed in **Table 1**, which is similar to other facelift techniques. Hematoma rates still remain at approximately 1.5%.[2,18,19] The most usual complications are earlobe revisions and temporal hairline scars. If secondary facelifts are necessary, then a full year must pass before any intervention.

SUPPLEMENTARY DATA

Supplementary data related to this article can be found online at https://doi.org/10.1016/j.cps.2019.06.003.

REFERENCES

1. Baker DC. Lateral SMASectomy, plication, and short-scar facelifts: indications and techniques. Clin Plast Surg 2008;35:533–50.
2. Baker DC, Levine SM. Lateral SMASectomy and facelift. In: Azzizzadeh B, Murphy M, Johnson C, et al, editors. Master techniques in facial rejuvenation. 2nd edition. Canada: Elsevier; 2018. p. 211–8.
3. Baker DC. Lateral SMASectomy. In: Neligan P, editor. Plastic surgery, vol. 2, 3rd edition. China: Elsevier; 2012. p. 232–7.
4. Baker DC. Short-scar rhytidectomy. In: Nahai F, editor. The art of aesthetic surgery: principles and techniques, vol. 2, 2nd edition. St. Louis (MO): QMP; 2011. p. 1436–70.
5. Baker DC. Deep dissection rhytidectomy: a plea for caution. Plast Reconstr Surg 1994;93(7):1498–9.
6. Baker DC, Conley J. Avoiding facial nerve injuries in rhytidectomy. Anatomical variations and pitfalls. Plast Reconstr Surg 1979;64:781–95.
7. Baker DC. Lateral SMASectomy. Plast Reconstr Surg 1997;100:509–13.
8. Baker DC. Lateral SMASectomy. Semin Plast Surg 2002;16:417–22.
9. Mitz V, Peyronie M. The superficial musculoaponeurotic system (SMAS) in the parotid and cheek area. Plast Reconstr Surg 1976;58(1):80–8.
10. Baker DC. Minimal incision rhytidectomy (short scar face lift) with lateral SMASectomy: evolution and application. Aesthet Surg J 2001;21:14–26.
11. Baker DC. Minimal incision rhytidectomy (short scar face lift) with lateral SMASectomy: operating strategies. Aesthet Surg J 2001;21:68–80.
12. Baker DC. Rhytidectomy with lateral SMASectomy. Facial Plast Surg 2000;16(3):209–13.
13. Alpert BS, Baker DC, Hamra ST, et al. Identical twin face lifts with differing techniques: a 10-year follow-up. Plast Reconstr Surg 2009;123:1025–36.
14. Ivy EJ, Lorenc ZP, Aston SJ. Is there a difference? A prospective study comparing lateral and standard SMAS face lifts with extended SMAS and composite rhytidectomies. Plast Reconstr Surg 1996;98(7):1135–43.
15. Camirand A, Doucet J. A comparison between parallel hairline incisions and perpendicular incisions when performing a facelift. Plast Reconstr Surg 1997;99(1):10–5.
16. Guerrero-Santos J, Espaillat L, Morales F. Muscular lift in cervical rhytidoplasty. Plast Reconstr Surg 1974;54(2):127–31.
17. Pelle-Ceravolo M, Angelini M, Silvi E. Treatment of anterior neck aging without a submental approach: lateral skin-plastysma displacement, a new and proven technique for platysma bands and skin laxity. Plast Reconstr Surg 2017;139:308–21.
18. Baker DC, Stefani W, Chiu ES. Reducing the incidence of hematoma requiring surgical evacuation following male rhytidectomy: a 30-year review of 985 cases. Plast Reconstr Surg 2005;116:1973–85.
19. Baker DC, Chiu ES. Bedside treatment of early acute rhytidectomy hematomas. Plast Reconstr Surg 2005;115(7):2119–22.

The Extended Superficial Musculoaponeurotic System

Ali H. Charafeddine, MD[a], James E. Zins, MD[b],*

KEYWORDS

• Facelift • SMAS • Facial rejuvenation

KEY POINTS

- Subcutaneous dissection should proceed under direct vision, creating a homogenous skin flap and leaving appropriate amount of fat on the superficial musculoaponeurotic system (SMAS).
- Skin and SMAS are separately raised, posing a technical challenge in the secondary facelift as well as thin patients.
- Release of the zygomatic and masseteric cutaneous ligaments is key in SMAS mobilization, with attention to the facial nerve branches running in close proximity to the ligaments.
- The great auricular nerve territory should be marked to avoid injury to this nerve.
- Exploration of the subplatysmal neck space is necessary in most patients.

INTRODUCTION

The mid 1970s marked the beginnings of modern facelift surgery. At that time the facelift operation evolved from wide skin undermining to an operation involving manipulation of the superficial fascia. This was in large part due to the works of Skoog, Mitz, and Peyronie and later Hamra and others. Conceptually superficial musculoaponeurotic system (SMAS) tightening acted as the vehicle to reposition facial fat and restore facial contour. The skin is then redraped under minimal tension.

The description of the sub-SMAS dissection plane and its importance in facial rejuvenation led to the development of the different strategies of SMAS elevation and reanchoring, which include the high-SMAS, the extended SMAS, the deep plane, and composite lifts. All these techniques have their advantages and disadvantages, and they all have shown good results. The key to a consistent excellent facial rejuvenation result does not depend on the technique used but rather on the tailoring of the operation to the aesthetic needs of the patient, which is achieved by a thorough preoperative examination.

HISTORY

Skoog[1] pioneered the era of modern facelift surgery by introducing the Skoog facelift. This entails minimal skin undermining and then a sub-SMAS flap in the cheek and a subplatysmal flap in the neck. This musculofascial flap was redraped along a cephaloposterior vector of pull. Once Mitz and Peyronie[2] described the SMAS as a separate unit, skin undermining and SMAS elevation gained worldwide popularity. Furnas,[3] in 1989, described the retaining ligaments of the face, which led to a better understanding of the aging-induced changes in the face.

In the late 90s, Coleman[4] popularized the concept of structural fat grafting, and later Rohrich and Pessa[5–7] described the fat compartments of the face. Many studies demonstrated the

Disclosures: The authors have nothing to disclose.
[a] Center for Plastic & Reconstructive Surgery, 5333 McAuley Drive, Suite 5001, Ypsilanti, MI 48197, USA;
[b] Department of Plastic Surgery, Cleveland Clinic, 9500 Euclid Avenue, A60, Cleveland, OH 44195, USA
* Corresponding author.
E-mail address: Zinsj@ccf.org

Clin Plastic Surg 46 (2019) 533–546
https://doi.org/10.1016/j.cps.2019.05.002

importance of facial fat in facial aging and the techniques used to restore it.[8-11] The concept of lift and fill[12] currently dominates the principles of facial rejuvenation, which includes (1) lifting or manipulating the SMAS and skin in different vectors of rejuvenation and (2) filling the fat compartments.

PHYSICAL EXAMINATION

A thorough preoperative physical examination is of paramount importance (**Fig. 1**). Particular attention is paid to the following points:

- Age, skin quality, and elasticity.
- Fitzpatrick classification of the skin.
- Horizontal thirds and vertical fifths of the face.
- Position of the brows and assessment if brow lift is needed as an adjunct procedure (Brow lift surgery is beyond the scope of this article.).
- Assess the upper and lower eyelids and point out any aging changes in these areas that would not be addressed by the facelift procedure alone.
- Contour changes happening secondary to the aging process: nasojugal groove, palpebral malar groove, nasolabial folds, marionette lines, jowls, jawline irregularities, neck platysma banding, and cervicomental angle changes.
- Degree of soft tissue deflation.
- Bony support in the malar area, zygomatic arch, and bigonial width.
- Degree of perioral rhytids.
- Upper lip length and assessment if an adjunct lip lift is needed.

ANATOMIC CONSIDERATIONS
A Design in Layers

The face is composed of concentric, cylindrical layers. In the concentric layered design of the face, deep to the skin is the superficial fascia or SMAS, which invests the muscles of facial expression.

It is crucial for the plastic surgeon planning a facelift operation to understand the details of the three-dimensional facial anatomy. The deepest concentric layer is the deep fascia or parotidomasseteric fascia (PMF), which covers the facial nerve branches proximally, the parotid duct, buccal fat pad, and the facial artery and vein more distally.[13] The reason why a sub-SMAS dissection can be performed safely is because facial nerve branches lie deep to the SMAS and deep to the PMF until the dissection reaches the retaining ligaments. At this time, the facial nerve branches pass from deep fascia to a sub-SMAS location to innervate their target muscles.

The Superficial Musculoaponeurotic System

The SMAS layer continues as the platysma in the neck, the frontalis muscle in the forehead, and the superficial temporal fascia in the temple area. The deep fascia continues as the deep cervical fascia in the neck, the deep temporal fascia in the temple area, and the periosteum in the region of the forehead/scalp.[13]

The Retaining Ligaments and Related Nerves

The retaining ligaments (**Fig. 2**) play a critical role in providing stability in the anterior/mobile portion of the face. They can originate from bone (zygomatic cutaneous ligaments, mandibular osteocutaneous ligaments) or from confluences of the deeper and superficial fascia (the masseteric cutaneous ligaments).[14] The release of these ligaments during SMAS elevation permits mobilization of the SMAS and the soft tissue distal to the retaining ligaments. Release of the retaining ligaments is done with care as the facial nerve branches run in the vicinity of these ligaments. Of interest in the

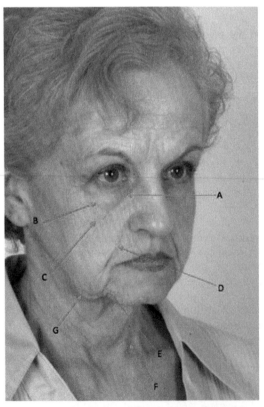

Fig. 1. Signs of aging in a 63-year-old woman. (A) Tear trough deformity. (B) Palpebromalar groove. (C) Loss of volume in the cheek. (D) Nasolabial folds. (E) Marionette lines. (F) Platysmal band. (G) Jowl formation.

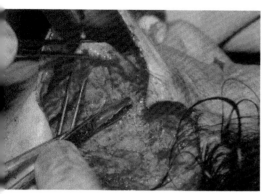

Fig. 2. Left side of a facelift dissection. The SMAS has been raised (lifted up by forceps). The Surgeon has his scissors behind the major zygomatic cutaneous ligament.

extended SMAS operation is the relationship be tween the zygomatic nerve branches (superior and inferior) with the major zygomatic cutaneous ligaments and the upper masseteric cutaneous ligaments. The upper branch of the zygomatic nerve is found in our cadaver dissections to be always deep to the zygomatic major muscle, whereas the lower branch passes in the direct vicinity of the upper masseteric cutaneous ligament.[15] This anatomy creates a safe passageway between the main zygomatic cutaneous ligament and the upper masseteric cutaneous ligament.

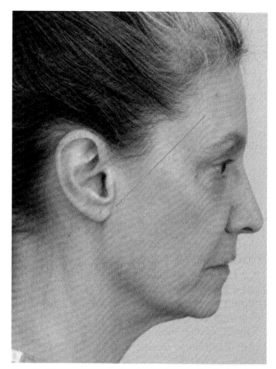

Fig. 3. The course of the frontal branch of the facial nerve as described by Pitanguy (*Blue line*).

The frontal branch of the facial nerve

The course of the frontal branch of the facial nerve was described by Pitanguy along a line starting 0.5 cm inferior to the tragus to a point 1.5 cm above the lateral brow[16] (**Fig. 3**). It usually corresponds to the middle third of the zygomatic arch (**Fig. 4**). The frontal branch lies deep to the SMAS as well as deep to the parotidomasseteric fascia (PMF) as it crosses the arch and is therefore deep and relatively out of harms' way. This anatomy becomes handy for the surgeon planning to raise an SMAS flap during a facelift. This anatomy is also essential when planning to anchor the SMAS flap after it is elevated.

PERIOPERATIVE PLANNING
Anesthesia and Prepping

This operation can be done under general anesthesia as well as under sedation with local anesthesia. Modern facelifts with SMAS flaps and adjunct procedures (eyelids, brow lift, lasers, or chemical peels) often require a prolonged operating time. The senior author described an anesthesia/prepping technique that assures safe intubation and ready access to the entire face. It has been tested in more than 400 cases with no

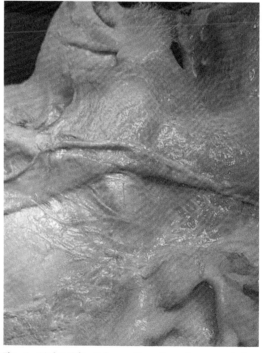

Fig. 4. Right side cadaver dissection. Arrow pointing to frontal branch of the facial nerve as it crosses the middle third of the zygomatic arch.

airway-related problems or other complications[17] (**Fig. 5**):

1. The face and entire head are prepped. We do not cover the hair, as those drapes commonly fall off during the operation.
2. Endotracheal intubation with a fiber reinforced tube (intraoral rather than intranasal) is used and wire fixed to the lower dentition with a single 26 wire.
3. The fiber reinforced tube is brought over the head cephalad rather than toward the neck. It can be moved down to the chin when the surgeon starts an adjunct procedurelike such as brow lift or eyelid surgery. The fiber reinforcement prevents kinking that can happen with nonreinforced tubes. The tube is connected to the anesthesia machine using a straight connector. It rests on a metal "christmas tree" (see **Fig. 5**).
4. When draping, a sterile stockinet is placed on the entire tube and christmas tree, thus preventing a breach of sterility.
5. An infiltration solution of 0.5% lidocaine and 1:200,000 epinephrine is injected subcutaneously in the side of the face that is started with. The authors believe this provides, in addition to the anesthetic effect, good vasoconstriction that allows excellent visualization and yet minimize the rebound bleeding once the symptomatic effect wears off.[18,19]

SURGICAL TECHNIQUE
Principles

In all the sub-SMAS operations, the plane of dissection is similar. The difference is the extent of skin undermining. The operation starts in the

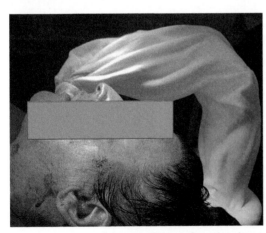

Fig. 5. Prepping and draping. The reinforced endotracheal tube is brought cephalad and rests on a "christmas tree."

subcutaneous plane, then under the SMAS at varying points, and once the zygomaticus major muscle is reached, the dissection goes in the subcutaneous plane again. The benefit of the extended SMAS when compared with Hamra's deep plane operation is that the vector of pull can be different between the skin and the SMAS. The SMAS pull is vertical while the skin pull is horizontal. The disadvantage is that the SMAS thins distally. Therefore, the risk of SMAS tearing is real, highlighting the technical challenge of the operation. In the deep plane or composite facelift, the SMAS is left attached to the skin for a much greater distance and the risk of tearing is thus negligible.[20–23] Regardless of the sub-SMAS procedure performed, release of the major zygomatic and upper masseteric cutaneous ligaments is critical to medial soft tissue mobilization.

Incisions

The senior author has used an anterior hairline incision in the temple area for over 35 years. This incision is carried from the preauricular area horizontally along the sideburn cheek junction and then vertically 3 to 4 mm within the anterior temporal hairline. This protects the hairline position, avoids injury to the superficial temporal artery, and hides the scar within the hair.

The preauricular incision is placed in the posttragal location in primary facelifts. When performing a secondary facelift, the previous incisions are used. In patients with a small delicate tragus, a pretragal incision may be considered to avoid any postoperative distortion. Men are treated similar to women.

The posterior preauricular incision in primary facelifts is placed high on the ear cartilage (1 cm above the posterior auricular sulcus), with the most cephalad part corresponding to the location of the root of the helix anteriorly (Feldman's touch point).[19] The incision in carried parallel and along the posterior hairline. When the distal end of the incision is reached, the incision is taken into the hair bearing skin to avoid detection. The caudal extension of this incision depends on the amount of excess skin in the neck that will be excised, keeping in mind that the vector of pull in this location is horizontal.

Skin Undermining

A homogenous skin flap is raised under direct vision using short curved iris scissors. It is necessary to leave a layer of fat on the SMAS as described by Stuzin, as this will help creating a robust SMAS flap.[13] It is not advisable to perform the subcutaneous dissection with the quick tunneling/undermining technique, as the surgeon will have no control on the homogeneity of the skin flap. Raising the flap too thick weakens the SMAS and may lead to tearing. Raising it too thin may compromise skin vascularization.

The subcutaneous dissection stops as the orbicularis muscle is reached in the temporal region, the malar eminence in the cheek, and past the marionette lines to release the mandibular osteocutaneous ligaments in the lower face. The subcutaneous dissection should only cross the nasolabial folds in selected patients with deep creases. Keeping in mind that every patient has different amount of excess skin and facial aging process, the extent of subcutaneous dissection is best planned in the perioperative area while marking the patient in an upright position.

As the surgeon approaches the territory of the great auricular nerve, a vertical line is marked along the middle of the lobule and perpendicular to Frankfurt's horizontal plane. Another line extends posteriorly at 30 degree[24] (**Fig. 6**). Injury to this nerve often resolves but entrapment can lead to distressful and painful neuromas. Of note, McKinney's point is often used to help locate the great auricular nerve at a point 6.5 cm inferior to the external auditory canal at the mid-belly of the sternocleidomastoid muscle.[25] However, one drawback to McKinney's point is that injury to the great auricular nerve may happen well before this point is reached. Using a 30-degree angle encourages the surgeon to perform a superficial dissection in the area of the nerve.

Now that the danger zone of the great auricular nerve is marked, the skin dissection proceeds in the neck in a supraplatysma plane. All the supraplatysma fat is left attached to the skin flap in the neck. This dissection proceeds until the midline of the neck is reached. Of note the skin flap elevation over the jawline should be from above downward, leaving jowl fat on the SMAS and not on the skin flap. This allows the elevated SMAS to reposition subcutaneous fat back into the face (**Fig. 7**). The subcutaneous dissection in the neck proceeds until the platysma mandibular ligaments are released.

Superficial Musculoaponeurotic System Dissection

The surgeon palpates the inferior border of the zygomatic arch. This corresponds to a line drawn along the top of the external auditory canal and marks the upper border of the SMAS flap. The vertical border of the SMAS flap is marked next, 2 cm anterior to the tragus. The caudal end of this line stays 2 cm posterior to the gonial angle and anterior to the great auricular nerve territory. The surgeon starts the sub-SMAS dissection staying at the lower portion of the ear or earlobe. Here the SMAS is very "platysmaish," muscular, and easy to identify. The deep dissection superficial to the parotid capsule is also obvious. Dissection then extends medially and superiorly anterior to the

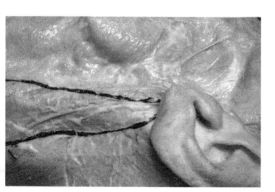

Fig. 6. Dissection of the left side of the face. Shown is the great auricular nerve (*arrow*) within the boundaries of Ozturk's triangle: The anterior limb is perpendicular to Frankfurt's horizontal and bisects the ear lobule. The posterior limb is drawn 30 degrees posteriorly.

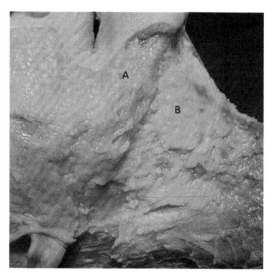

Fig. 7. Right side dissection of a fresh cadaver. (A) Jowl fat. (B) Supraplatysmal fat. While keeping all the supraplatysmal fat on the skin flap in the neck (B), the surgeon needs to pay careful attention not to proceed cephalad and raise the Jowl fat (A).

parotid gland where a thin fatty layer protects the parotid masseteric fascia. This fat should stay down on the fascia, thus protecting the facial nerve. As the surgeon is dissecting the SMAS flap superiorly, care should be taken to maintain the dissection at the lower edge of the zygomatic arch until the major zygomatic cutaneous ligaments and the upper masseteric cutaneous ligaments are released and the zygomaticus major (ZM) muscle is visualized. Once the ZM is reached, dissection proceeds superficial to it and follows a subcutaneous plane medially to the nasolabial fold. The surgeon will notice immediate release and easier cephalad mobilization of the SMAS once these ligaments are released. Once SMAS dissection is complete, the SMAS is sutured in a superior-vertical direction. Marking the trajectory of the frontal branch of the facial nerve avoids injury to this nerve during anchoring of the SMAS.

Next, an inferiorly base flap of SMAS is fashioned from the posterior (preauricular) edge of the SMAS; it is transposed posteriorly and sutured to the mastoid periosteum. This helps define the lower jaw border. Finally, careful assessment of the jowl fat and submandibular fat is performed. Fat at this location should be resected along and cephalad to the jawline to achieve a youthful facial shape.

Neck Management

A submental incision and anterior platysma surgery is indicated in almost all patients.[19,26] An incision is placed 1 cm posterior to the submental crease and dissection proceeds in the supraplatysmal plane. The submental dissection thus joins these 2 lateral dissections. Platysma cutaneous attachments adjacent to this incision are released under direct vision. The platysma is opened in the midline and the subplatysmal fat compartment is explored. Subplatysmal fat resection should leave fat flush with the anterior digastric muscles and not any further (**Fig. 8**). This avoids the "cobra" deformity (submental hollowness resulting from excess fat resection from the subplatysmal plane). Defatting extends inferiorly to the thyroid cartilage. The platysma is imbricated from the chin to thyroid cartilage. A second raw from the thyroid cartilage to the chin is then performed.[19]

Closure

Careful attention to hemostasis lowers the risk of hematoma formation. A bipolar cautery device is used for this purpose. Bipolar rather than

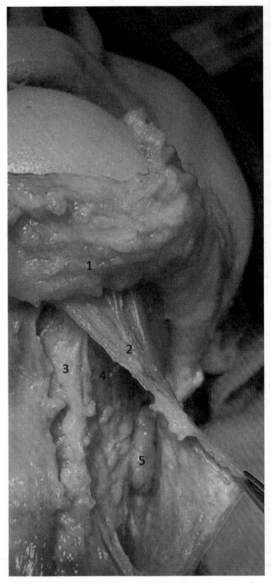

Fig. 8. Cadaver dissection showing the structures that contribute to the aging process in the neck. (1) Supraplatysmal fat (raised cephalad). (2) Left platysma muscle. (3) Subplatysmal fat. (4) Left digastric muscle. (5) Left submandibular glands.

unipolar cautery significantly reduces facial nerve neuropraxia as well as results in less serous drainage. During hemostasis, the patient's blood pressure is brought to the same level it was in the preoperative holding area. The excess skin is resected using a Zins Facelift Marker (Accurate Surgical & Scientific Instruments, Corp., Westbury, NY, USA) (**Fig. 9**) as a guide, and closure proceeds after drains are placed in the subcutaneous plane in the neck.

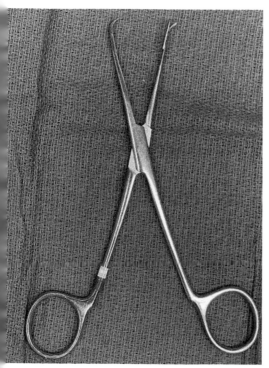

Fig. 9. Zins Facelift Marker. (Accurate Surgical & Scientific Instruments, Corp., Westbury, NY, USA; ASSI product number ASSI.ATK64526).

A 3-0 prolene suture is placed at the level of the root of the helix and another one is placed at the most cephalad part of the postauricular skin flap.

The authors use 5-0 (temporal hairline) and 6-0 (periauricular and submental incision) fast absorbing sutures for the skin closure. Subcutaneous deep dermal sutures with 4-0 monocryl are used in addition in the posterior auricular incisions and submental incision.

At the end of closure, the surgeon makes certain that the suction on the drains is maintained. The hair is washed with soap and water after extubation. A minimal soft dressing is used. The patient is invariably seen the next morning. Drains are generally removed in 24 hours.

Patients should have the preauricular sutures removed routinely 5 to 6 days after surgery. Standardized postoperative photographs are taken 4, 6, and 12 months after surgery (**Figs. 10–14**).

COMPLICATIONS
Early Complications

An acutely expanding hematoma needs an immediate return to the operating room to prevent skin flap compromise and/or airway problems.[27,28] A small hematoma discovered in the postanesthesia care unit can be safely drained at the bedside.[29] A missed small hematoma can lead to fibrosis and thus contour abnormalities.

The literature reports 1% to 11% incidence of hematoma formation after facelift surgery.[30,31] The most common risk factors for hematoma formation are aspirin and aspirin-like products (including herbal supplements, nonsteroidal antiinflammatory drugs, garlic supplements, vitamins), male gender, history of hypertension, and anterior platysmaplasty.[29,30,32,33] Perioperative hypertension has a direct correlation with hematoma formation. Patients with postoperative hypertension are aggressively treated according to protocol.[34,35] A particularly important point is to increase the blood pressure to normal levels at the time of closure to make sure hemostasis is well achieved. The use of dilute epinephrine (1:400,000), meticulous hemostasis, and increasing the blood pressure to normal or supranormal levels at the time of closure will reduce the likelihood of hematoma.[18] A second look or postponing closure of the first side until the second side is completed leads to a reduced epinephrine effect.[36]

Permanent facial nerve injury after a facelift is a feared but rare complication. It has been reported to be less than 1% in the literature, but this may be underreported.[37] The marginal mandibular and frontal branches are at risk due to the lack of cross-innervation that the other branches of the facial nerve have.[32,33] At times patients wake up after a facelift with an asymmetric smile, most commonly associated with the infiltration of local anesthesia, and commonly resolves on postop day one. An expectant management is usually sufficient.[38]

Long-Term Complications

- Pixie ear deformity
- Scarring after skin necrosis.
- Deformity of the tragus.
- Misplacement of the hairline (temporal and posterior auricular).
- Contour irregularities (missed hematomas or seromas)
- Recurrence of platysmal bands.

SUMMARY

In summary, the anatomic basis of the aging landmarks of the face are now well understood. The

540

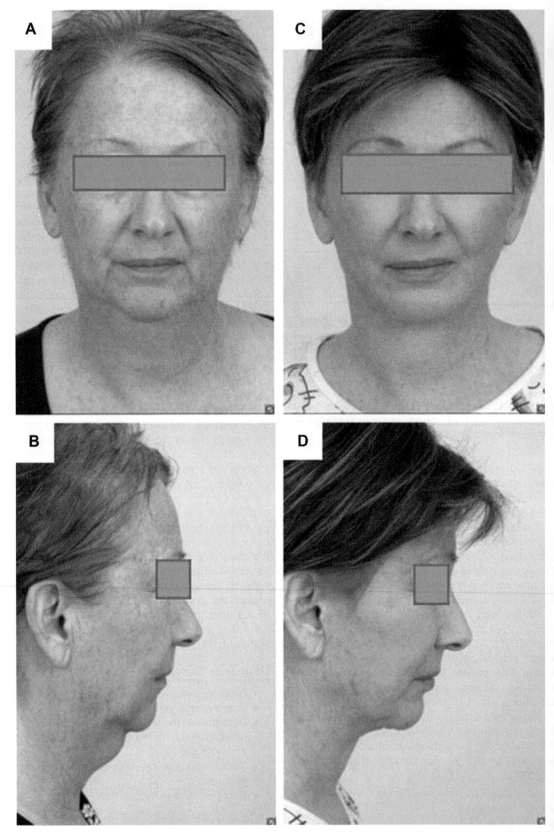

Fig. 10. A 63-year-old woman. (*A*) Preoperative anterior view and (*B*) lateral view. (*C*) Anterior and (*D*) lateral views 15 months after extended SMAS facelift, neck lift with anterior lipectomy and corset platysmaplasty. The patient received a full face fractional laser 6 months postoperatively.

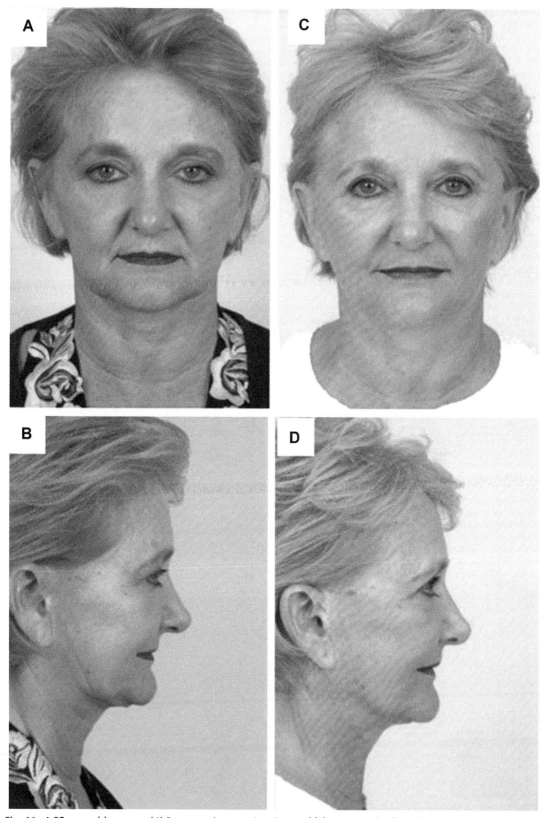

Fig. 11. A 58-year-old woman. (*A*) Preoperative anterior view and (*B*) preoperative lateral view presenting for a secondary facelift operation 6 years after her first extended SMAS procedure. (*C*) Anterior and (*D*) lateral views 6 years after secondary extended SMAS facelift, anterior neck lipectomy, corset platysmaplasty, and an endoscopic brow lift.

542

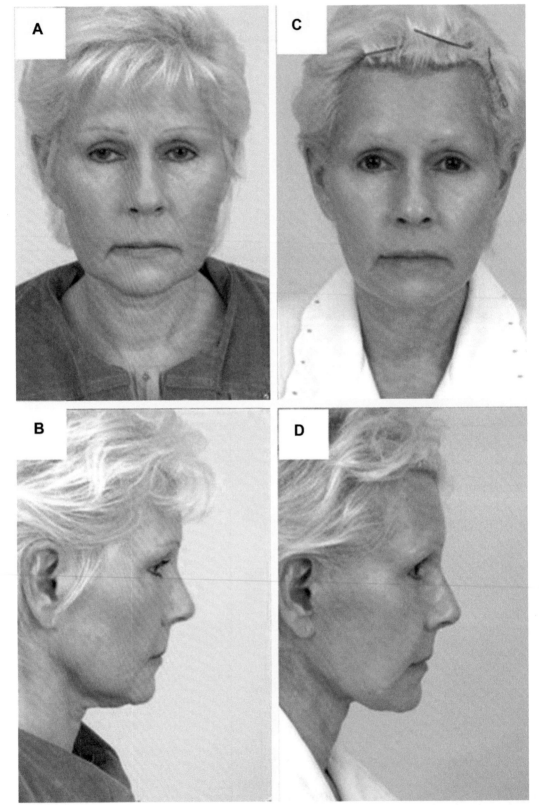

Fig. 12. A 58-year-old woman. (*A*) Anterior and (*B*) lateral views preoperatively. (*C*) Anterior and (*D*) lateral views 2 years after extended SMAS facelift, corset platysmaplasty, anterior neck lipectomy, lip lift, and fat injections into temples, cheeks, upper and lower lips. One month postoperatively the patient received bilateral upper eyelid ptosis repair and blepharoplasty.

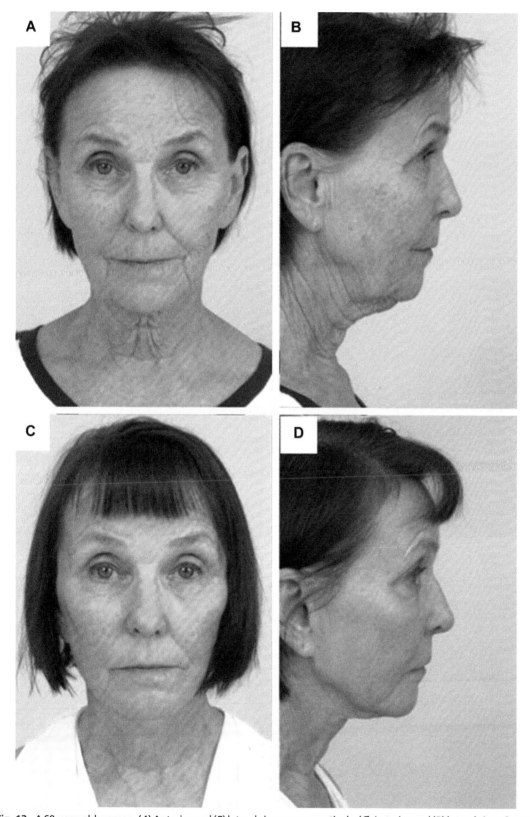

Fig. 13. A 69-year-old woman. (*A*) Anterior and (*B*) lateral views preoperatively. (*C*) Anterior and (*D*) lateral views 3 years after extended SMAS facelift, corset platysmaplasty, anterior neck lipectomy, and perioral phenol croton oil peel.

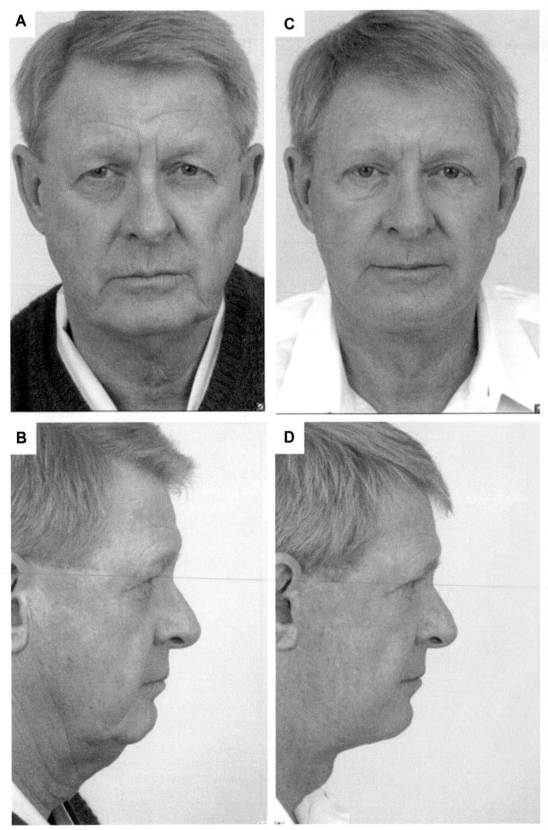

Fig. 14. A 64-year-old male patient. (*A*) Anterior and (*B*) lateral views preoperatively. (*C*) Anterior and (*D*) lateral views 3 years after extended SMAS facelift, corset platysmaplasty, and anterior neck lipectomy.

goals of aesthetic facial rejuvenation surgery can be tailored to appropriately address separately the changes that happen with the aging process.

The deflation of volume is addressed with strategic transfer of fat into the well-described fat compartments, and the extended SMAS lift (as well as other SMAS manipulation techniques) is a powerful method to correct the descent of the soft tissues.

One should not underestimate the power of the adjunct procedures that address the skin layer, whether mechanical (microneedling), chemical (phenol or other peels), and light-based (laser) modalities.

REFERENCES

1. Skoog T. New methods and refinements. In: Skoog T, editor. Plastic surgery. 1st edition. Stokholm (Sweden): Almgrist and wicksell International; 1974. p. 300–30.
2. Mitz V, Peyronie M. The superficial musculoaponeurotic system (SMAS) in the parotid and cheek area. PlastReconstr Surg 1976;58(1):80–8.
3. Furnas DW. The retaining ligaments of the cheek. PlastReconstr Surg 1989;83(1):11–6.
4. Coleman SR. Structural fat grafting. AesthetSurg J 1998;18(386):388.
5. Rohrich RJ, Pessa JE, Ristow B. The youthful cheek and the deep medial fat compartment. PlastReconstr Surg 2008;121:2107–12.
6. Rohrich RJ, Pessa JE. The fat compartments of the face: anatomy and clinical implications for cosmetic surgery. PlastReconstr Surg 2007;119:2219–27 [discussion: 2228–31].
7. Rohrich RJ, Arbique GM, Wong C, et al. The anatomy of suborbicularis fat: implications for periorbital rejuvenation. PlastReconstr Surg 2009;124:946–51.
8. Gierloff M, Stöhring C, Buder T, et al. Aging changes of the midfacial fat compartments: a computed tomographic study. PlastReconstr Surg 2012;129:263–73.
9. Gosain AK, Klein MH, Sudhakar PV, et al. A volumetric analysis of soft-tissue changes in the aging midface using high-resolution MRI: implications for facial rejuvenation. PlastReconstr Surg 2005;115:1143–52 [discussion: 1153–55].
10. Bucky LP, Kanchwala SK. The role of autologous fat and alternative fillers in the aging face. PlastReconstr Surg 2007;120(Suppl):89S–97S.
11. Gierloff M, Stöhring C, Buder T, et al. The subcutaneous fat compartments in relation to aesthetically important facial folds and rhytides. J PlastReconstrAesthet Surg 2012;65:1292–7.
12. Rohrich RJ, Ghavami A, Constantine FC, et al. Lift-and-Fill face lift. PlastReconstr Surg 2014;133(6):756e–67e.
13. Stuzin JM, Baker TJ, Gordon HL. The relationship of the superficial and deep facial fascias: relevance to rhytidectomy and aging. PlastReconstr Surg 1992;89(3):441–9 [discussion: 450–1].
14. Mendelson BC, Muzaffar AR, Adams WP. Surgical anatomy of the midcheek and malar mounds. PlastReconstr Surg 2002;110:885–96.
15. Alghoul M, Bitik O, McBride J, et al. Relationship of the zygomatic facial nerve to the retaining ligaments of the face: the Sub-SMAS danger zone. PlastReconstr Surg 2013;131(2):245e–52e.
16. Pitanguy I, Ramos S. The frontal branch of the facial nerve: the importance of its variations in Face lifting. PlastReconstrSurg 1966;(38):352–6.
17. Dobryansky M, Morrison CM, Zins JE. Patient draping and endotracheal tube positioning during facelift surgery. Ann Plast Surg 2009;63(1):9–10.
18. Swanson E. Evaluation of face lift skin perfusion and epinephrine effect using laser fluorescence imaging. PlastReconstrSurg Glob Open 2015;3(8):e484.
19. Feldman JJ. Neck lift my way. PlastReconstr Surg 2014;134(6):1173–83.
20. Stuzin JM, Baker TJ, Gordon HL, et al. Extended SMAS dissection as an approach to midface rejuvenation. ClinPlast Surg 1995;22(2):295–311. Available at: http://www.ncbi.nlm.nih.gov/pubmed/7634739.
21. Mendelson BC. Extended sub-SMAS dissection and cheek elevation. ClinPlast Surg 1995;22(2):325–39. Available at: http://www.ncbi.nlm.nih.gov/pubmed/7634741.
22. Stuzin JM. MOC-PSSM CME article: face lifting. PlastReconstr Surg 2008;121(1 Suppl):1–19.
23. Stuzin JM. Restoring facial shape in face lifting: the role of skeletal support in facial analysis and midface soft-tissue repositioning. PlastReconstr Surg 2007;119(1):362–76, 378.
24. Ozturk CN, Ozturk C, Huettner F, et al. A failsafe method to avoid injury to the great auricular nerve. AesthetSurg J 2014;34(1):16–21.
25. McKinney P, Katrana DJ. Prevention of injury to the great auricular nerve during rhytidectomy. PlastReconstr Surg 1980;66(5):675–9.
26. Feldman JJ. Surgical anatomy of the neck. In: Necklift. 1st edition. Stuttgart (Germany): Thieme; 2006. p. 106–13.
27. Schnur PL, Weinzweig J. A second look at the second-look technique in face lifts. PlastReconstr Surg 1995;96(7):1724–6. Available at:http://www.ncbi.nlm.nih.gov/pubmed/7480299.
28. Maricevich MA, Adair MJ, Maricevich RL, et al. Facelift complications related to median and peak blood pressure evaluation. AesthetPlast Surg 2014;38(4):641–7.
29. Grover R, Jones BM, Waterhouse N. The prevention of haematoma following rhytidectomy: a review of

1078 consecutive facelifts. Br J Plast Surg 2001; 54(6):481–6.

30. Jones BM, Grover R. Avoiding hematoma in cervicofacialrhytidectomy: a personal 8-year quest. Reviewing 910 patients. PlastReconstr Surg 2004;113:381–7, 390.

31. Jones B, Grover R. Reducing complications in cervicofacialrhytidectomy by tumescent infiltrate.A comparative trial of 678 consecutive facelifts. PlastReonstr Surg 2004;131:121e.

32. Gupta V, Winocour J, Shi H, et al. Preoperative risk factors and complication rates in facelift: analysis of 11,300 patients. AesthetSurg J 2015;36:1–13.

33. Baker DC, Aston SJ, Guy CL, et al. The male rhytidectomy. PlastReconstr Surg 1977;60(4):514–22. Available at: http://www.ncbi.nlm.nih.gov/pubmed/909960.

34. Beer GM, Goldscheider E, Weber A, et al. Prevention of acute hematoma after face-lifts. AesthetPlast Surg 2010;34(4):502–7.

35. Ramanadham SR, Mapula S, Costa C, et al. Evolution of hypertension management in face lifting in 1089 patients: optimizing safety and outcomes. PlastReconstr Surg 2015;135(4):1037–43.

36. Baker DC, Stefani WA, Chiu ES. Reducing the incidence of hematoma requiring surgical evacuation following male rhytidectomy: a 30-year review of 985 cases. PlastReconstr Surg 2005;116(7): 1973–85 [discussion: 1986–7].

37. Matarasso A, Elkwood A, Rankin M, et al. National plastic surgery survey: face lift techniques and complications. PlastReconstr Surg 2000;106(5): 1185–95 [discussion: 1196]. Available at:http://www.ncbi.nlm.nih.gov/pubmed/11039390.

38. Roostaeian J, Rohrich RJ, Stuzin JM. Anatomical considerations to prevent facial nerve injury. PlastReconstr Surg 2015;135(5):1318–27.

The Minimal Access Cranial Suspension Lift

Mustafa Chopan, MD, Patrick J. Buchanan, MD, Bruce A. Mast, MD*

KEYWORDS

• Facelift • Rhytidectomy • MACS • Facial rejuvenation • Facial aging

KEY POINTS

• The minimal access cranial suspension (MACS) facelift provides a short scar with vertical resuspension of the soft tissue without the need to formally open the neck.
• This technique is ideal for patients with mild to moderate skin laxity without significant lipodystrophy of the neck region.
• In properly selected patients, excellent facial rejuvenation is achieved, affording a quicker recovery, reduction in operative time, and the potential for concurrent nonfacial procedures.

 Video content accompanies this article at http://www.plasticsurgery.theclinics.com.

INTRODUCTION

Facial aging is a multifactorial process characterized by anatomic elements affected by time and the environment.[1–3] Key among these are the following:

• Descent and volumetric loss of the facial components
• Increased skin laxity
• Increased laxity of retaining ligaments
• Actinic damage
• Lipoatrophy
• Bony depletion

The principles of facial rejuvenation are centered on the correction of these composite tissue alterations. As such, modern facial rejuvenation has evolved into a multimodal approach consisting of skin resurfacing, soft tissue fillers, neuromodulators, and surgical interventions. A fundamental understanding of the anatomic changes seen with facial aging is paramount in selecting the ideal procedure for facial rejuvenation.

Historically, surgical facial rejuvenation consisted of discontinuous elliptical skin excisions to help remove skin creases and tighten the skin. Indeed, the term rhytidectomy arose from the essence of the procedure and removal of skin wrinkles. Technical advancements, such as wide undermining and superficial musculoaponeurotic system (SMAS) manipulation, were made possible as the understanding of facial anatomy improved. Since the initial descriptions of skin-tightening procedures, various approaches and techniques have developed to address more than just the removal of wrinkles. Each procedure differs in nuance with regard to plane of dissection and handling of laminar structures. The established procedures of today are used with some variation of incisions to achieve maximal skin resection, elevation of the SMAS to restore volume, and autologous fat grafting or synthetic fillers to correct soft tissue atrophy.[4–6]

Over the past decade, there has been greater interest in minimally invasive procedures for facial rejuvenation. In particular, the minimal access

Disclosure Statement: The authors have nothing to disclose.
Department of Surgery, University of Florida College of Medicine, PO Box 100138, Gainesville, FL 32610-0138, USA
* Corresponding author.
E-mail address: bruce.mast@surgery.ufl.edu
🐦; @DrMChopan (M.C.); @DrPJBuchanan (P.J.B.); @GatorPlastSurg (B.A.M.)

Clin Plastic Surg 46 (2019) 547–557
https://doi.org/10.1016/j.cps.2019.06.005

cranial suspension (MACS) facelift is a minimally invasive procedure for facial rejuvenation first described by Tonnard and colleagues[7] in 2002. The procedure is a "short-scar" face and neck lift that uses a continuous preauricular and temporal incision with no extension into the postauricular sulcus, posterior scalp, nor cervical hairline. There is limited skin undermining, and the neck is not opened in a separate incision. The facial and neck soft tissues are elevated via SMAS and platysma plication/imbrication using looped, purse-string sutures, and the remaining excess skin is appropriately excised. The advantages of this technique include shorter operative times, quicker recovery, and less patient morbidity. In the right patient, and executed with sound surgical technique, this procedure can produce excellent results and a satisfied patient.

SURGICAL FOUNDATION OF THE MINIMAL ACCESS CRANIAL SUSPENSION FACELIFT

The MACS facelift addresses volume restoration and laxity by composite elevation of the deep facial structures using cranially fixated looped sutures and concomitant skin tightening. The essence of surgical facial rejuvenation is the correction of soft tissue descent with resuspension of descended tissues to structures that are less affected by the facial aging process. In the MACS facelift, the SMAS and platysma are anchored to the deep fascia (either deep temporal or Lore fascia). The "minimal access" feature of this technique limits the incision to the temporal area and preauricular border. However, in cases of increased skin laxity, a retroauricular extension may be indicated.

The key elements of the MACS lift are the following:

- Skin incision without postauricular extension
- No opening of the neck
- Limited skin flap elevation
- SMAS plication via purse-string, looped sutures with superior fascial fixation
- Vertical skin vector tightening

As originally described by Tonnard and colleagues,[7–9] 2 obliquely oriented looped sutures are used in the cheek and a vertically oriented looped suture is used in the neck. The "extended-MACS" facelift adds another, third, looped purse-string suture in the malar region to resuspend the malar fat pad. This third suture has been abandoned by the senior author (B.A.M.) in favor of a broader single-looped suture in the cheek region to better accomplish midface and malar fat pad elevation.

The laminar anatomy of the face allows for the combined movement and elevation of the deep facial structures as a composite flap without surgical delamination. By capturing the platysma muscle below the angle of the mandible, the first vertical looped suture lifts the soft tissues in the neck. Similarly, the second, obliquely oriented cheek suture captures and lifts the soft tissues of the midcheek, the malar fat pad, and jowl. The skin is redraped in a vertically oriented fashion and excess tissue is appropriately excised.

The technique of using a purely vertical pull on the SMAS complex not only sheet-tightens and elevates the SMAS and underlying structures but also causes bunching of the soft tissues within the loop (referred to as "microimbrication"), which further aids in volume restoration in the aged/attenuated face. The neck lift is accomplished using the same continuous temporal and preauricular incision via the use of the vertical purse-string suture by virtue of its contiguous extension with the SMAS into the platysma. The vertical movement of the lateral platysma just inferior to the angle of the mandible extends to the anterior platysma, creating lifting and contouring of the entire width of the anterior neck. There is no open treatment of the neck with an anterior or "corset" platysmaplasty. Thus, the close relationship of the platysma and overlying skin is maintained, allowing the tissues to efficiently move together in the aponeurotic superficial plane.[10] Cervical liposuction is used when indicated.

PREOPERATIVE EVALUATION AND PATIENT SELECTION

An ideal approach to facial rejuvenation is holistic, because each patient is unique with respect to his or her aesthetic needs. Although surgery is an integral part of facial rejuvenation, ancillary procedures, such as fillers, laser therapy, neuromodulators, and medical skin care, can work synergistically to produce excellent results.

As in all potential patients being considered for surgical facial rejuvenation, various facial components require careful evaluation and planning. Facial nerve and muscular function, along with any asymmetries, should be noted before intervention. Skeletal support, such as chin or malar deficiency, should be addressed. The use of skin resurfacing, neurotoxins, and fillers before surgery are dependent on the patient's goals and objectives, combined with the unique findings of each individual. Similarly, the benefits of brow lift, blepharoplasty, and fat grafting in conjunction with, or separated from, the facelift should be fully assessed.

Specific to an MACS lift, it is paramount to accurately assess the extent of cervicofacial laxity and neck adiposity to ensure proper choice of technique and success. Initial publications of the procedure as well as presentations and lectures advocated that the MACS facelift is an effective tool for virtually all patients seeking midface and lower-face/neck facial rejuvenation. After transitioning to a nearly exclusive practice of MACS facelifts, and with careful analysis of postoperative outcomes, the senior author (B.A.M.) identified limitations to the procedure.[11,12] The technique is not ideal for patients with severe facial skin laxity, because the looped sutures and vertical vector of skin excision lead to an increased incidence of skin pleating in the lateral periorbital region near the temporal hairline as well as along the lateral neck inferior to the lobule. Likewise, bulky necks treated with combined liposuction will often have excess cervical laxity inadequately corrected without the traditional facelift skin tightening and excision techniques (**Figs. 1** and **2**). Instead, those patients with notable cervical-facial skin excess or laxity would be best served with a conventional facelift. Thus, the MACS facelift is better suited for patients with mild to moderate skin laxity/

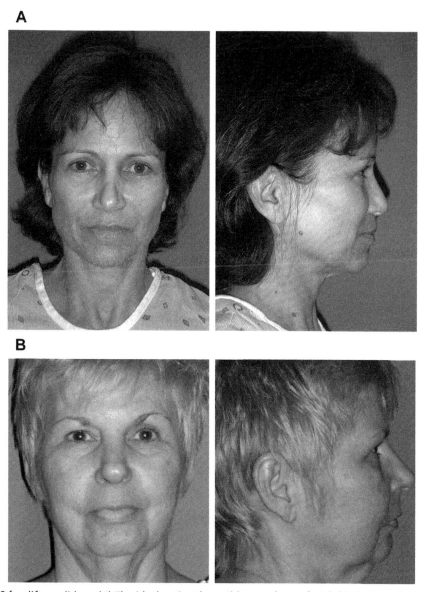

Fig. 1. MACS facelift candidacy. (*A*) The ideal patient has mild to moderate facial skin laxity and cervical lipodystrophy (frontal and lateral views). (*B*) Nonideal patients have excess facial skin laxity or, as pictured here, severe cervical lipodystrophy (frontal and lateral views).

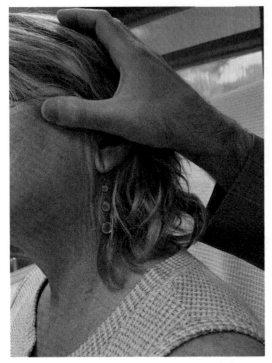

Fig. 2. Excess skin laxity can be appreciated upon simulating the vertical vector of tissue elevation preoperatively. If pleating of the skin at the lobule extending onto the neck, occurs, the patient is a poor candidate for MACS facelift.

excess and less cervical lipodystrophy. As such, younger, thinner patients and those who have not experienced massive weight loss are ideal candidates. Patients presenting for secondary or revision facelift are also candidates for the MACS lift dependent on the degree of recurrent skin

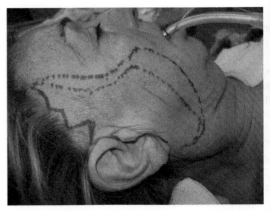

Fig. 4. Modifications to the MACS facelift. A zigzag incision is fashioned in the anterior scalp, and subcutaneous undermining can be further extended in patients with a greater degree of skin laxity (*anterior dotted line*).

laxity, which is often mild to moderate. The use of limited dissection and the purse-string plication of the SMAS provides the added advantage of avoiding potentially risky dissections in deeper planes.[13]

SURGICAL PROCEDURE

The incision is marked from the anterior temporal hairline, then posteriorly in a horizontal manner at the base of the sideburn, continued along the anterior upper auricular border, extending posterior to the tragus and the along the preauricular line, stopping at the lobule (**Fig. 3**). Alternatively, the temporal incision can be moved into the anterior scalp, as a zigzag incision line, while maintaining the horizontal incision along the sideburn (**Fig. 4**). The extent of flap elevation is marked, extending obliquely from the upper aspect of the temporal scalp past the lateral orbit, to over the

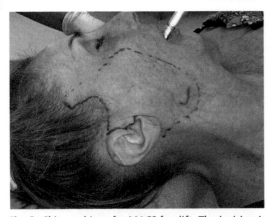

Fig. 3. Skin markings for MACS facelift. The incision is made along the temporal hairline and extends inferiorly along the preauricular border to the ear lobule. The dotted outline signifies the extent of subcutaneous undermining.

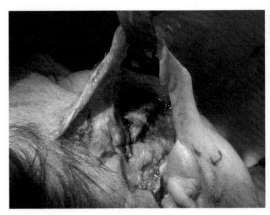

Fig. 5. Midface suture placement as outlined on the SMAS complex.

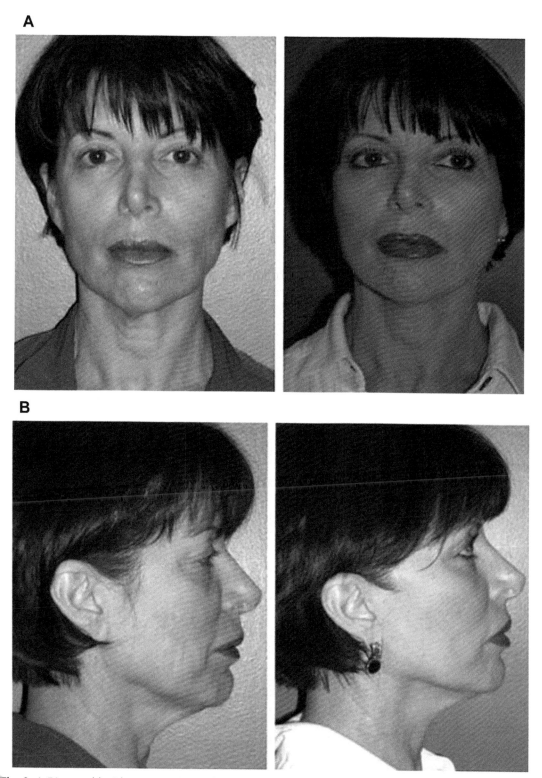

Fig. 6. A 54-year-old with preoperative and 9-month postoperative views following MACS facelift. (*A*) Frontal view. (*B*) Lateral view.

A

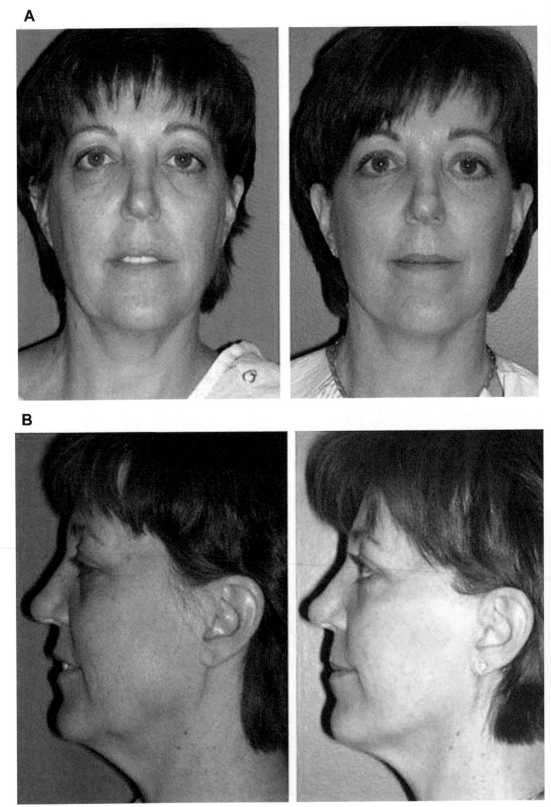

B

Fig. 7. A 54-year-old with facial changes associated with aging. Preoperative and 5-month postoperative photographs were obtained following MACS facelift and bilateral upper/lower blepharoplasties. (*A*) Frontal view. (*B*) Lateral view.

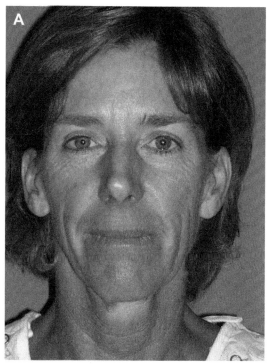

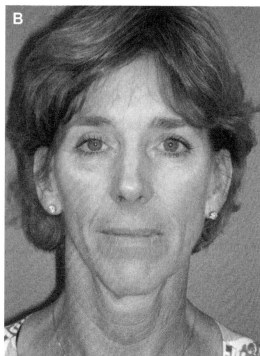

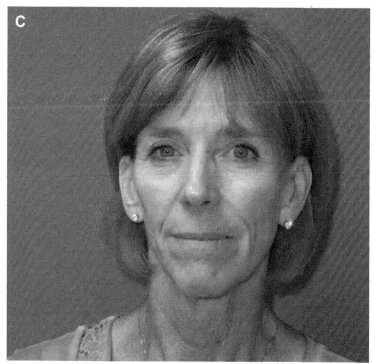

Fig. 8. (*A–C*) Anterior views of the MACS lift patient. (*A*) Preoperative view of a 59-year-old woman noting cervicofacial cutaneous laxity, deep nasolabial and labiomental folds, and rectangular facial morphology. (*B*) Two years after MACS lift: excellent cheek volume restoration, with correction of rectangular facial appearance to an angular morphology. (*C*) Nine years after MACS lift: cheek volume is retained, as is angular facial appearance.

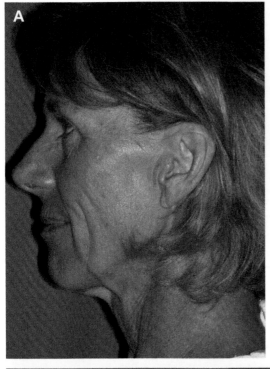

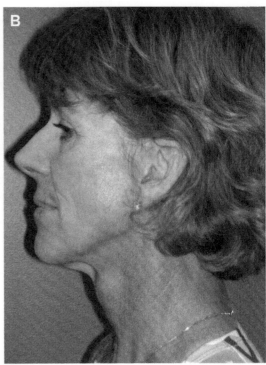

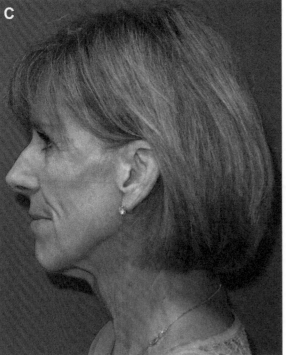

Fig. 9. (A–C) Lateral views of the MACS lift patient. (A) Preoperative view of a 59-year-old woman, noting prominent lower lid/cheek transition with cheek volume deficiency, deep nasolabial and labiomental folds, ill-defined mandibular contour, and cervical cutaneous laxity. (B) Two years after MACS lift: excellent smoothing of the lower lid/cheek transition with midface/cheek volume restoration, improvement of nasolabial and labiomental folds, and good definition of the mandibular contour. Cervical laxity is improved, but incompletely corrected centrally. (C) Nine years after MACS lift: excellent retention of lid/cheek transition, cheek volume, mandibular, and neck contouring. Recurrence of nasolabial and labiomental folds is noted, but still much improved from original preoperative appearance.

A

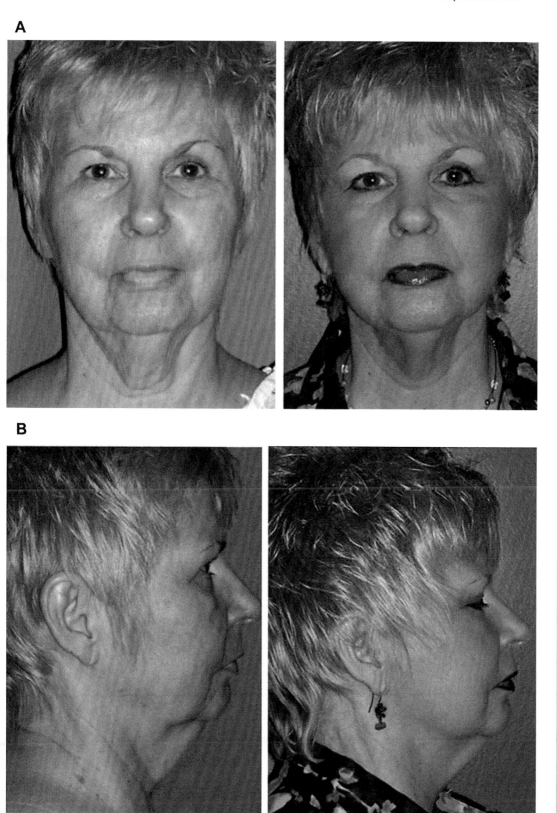

B

Fig. 10. Patient with excess cervical laxity and residual bulk following MACS facelift. (*A*) Frontal view. (*B*) Lateral view. This is an example of the limitations of the MACS lift. More thorough cervical rejuvenation would have occurred with a conventional facelift technique.

lateral malar prominence, then inferoposteriorly toward the mandibular angle extending to the upper neck near the angle, and then back upwards to the lobule. In patients with greater skin laxity, additional subcutaneous undermining is warranted to allow for further redraping of the skin (see **Fig. 4**). The incisions and subcutaneous plane beneath the skin flap are infiltrated with 0.5% lidocaine with 1:200,000 of epinephrine. After the appropriate time for hemostatic effect, the incision is created. The SMAS layer is identified, and the flap is elevated in the plane just superficial to the SMAS to the extent noted by the skin markings. Toward the scalp, the dissection is superficial to the temporoparietal fascia, whereas inferiorly, the plane continues superficial to the platysma.

After flap elevation and hemostasis, the deep temporal fascia is identified. This fascia is used as the anchoring point for the purse-string sutures. The SMAS is incised just inferior to the horizontal sideburn incision, at the inferior aspect of the zygoma. The superficial temporal artery and vein are identified and preserved. The dissection is carried down to the deep temporal fascia (Video 1). The dissection is continued anteriorly for the full length of the sideburn and superiorly to allow the anchoring suture and knot to be located as deeply as possible. The narrow, preauricular purse-string suture is then placed, beginning in the deep temporal fascia, continuing through the SMAS and making the looped turn 1 to 2 cm inferior to the angle of the mandible, incorporating the platysma. The suture is continued superiorly such that the loop is about 1.5 cm in width. Upon tightening and tying the knot, the neck and lower face are vertically recontoured (Videos 2 and 3). Next, the midface soft tissue is grasped atraumatically and pulled in the vector required for repositioning of the descended midfacial structures. The path of the purse-string placement is marked, after which the suture is placed (**Fig. 5**). Because of the broader nature of this purse-string, a third looped suture as described by Tonnard is not needed. The senior author (B.A.M.) prefers the use of a 2-0 nonabsorbable monofilament suture for the purse-string. The incised SMAS that provided access to the deep temporal fascia is reapproximated with absorbable suture. The skin flap is then retracted vertically, and further undermining/dissection of the flap is done as needed to correct any tethered points that prevent proper redraping. The skin flap is then advanced in a nearly vertical vector, incised and inset at the superior root of the helix. The lobule is then delivered by vertical inferior continuation of the lower aspect of the incision. The excess skin is marked and excised, and the flap is inset (Video 4).

When adjunctive facial procedures are performed, cervical liposuction and brow lift precede the MACS lift, whereas blepharoplasty is performed after completion of the MACS lift. The senior author (B.A.M.) most often performs a skin-only lower blepharoplasty using the skin-pinch technique. The limited lower blepharoplasty is made possible due to the elevation of the midface accomplished with the MACS lift, and the effect on the lower lid–check interface, which is additive for volume and skin redundancy. Because of the reduced time needed for this minimally invasive procedure, nonfacial procedures can safely be performed as well. Breast augmentation, mastopexy, mini-abdominoplasty, and trunk and abdominal liposuction are all procedures that have been performed concomitantly.

OUTCOMES

The MACS facelift is an effective and efficient technique in facial rejuvenation (**Figs. 6–9**). Patient satisfaction scores approach traditional facelift techniques (96%) with significantly less operative time (2.6 hours vs 4.1 hours).[12] To address other aspects of facial aging, ancillary facial procedures are often performed concomitantly, similar to conventional facelifts. As noted above, the diminished time required for an MACS facelift allows for significantly more concurrent nonfacial procedures compared with conventional techniques (23% vs 0%).[11] Complications are nearly equitable with regard to hematoma, infection, delayed wound healing, temporary paresis, or abnormal scarring. Nevertheless, there is a significantly higher incidence of postoperative skin pleating (submental, temporal, and periocular regions) in a certain cohort of MACS patients. Such patients are characterized with excess laxity and are often dissatisfied with the residual loose-tissue deformities, particularly in the cervical region (**Fig. 10**). The effect of the procedure appears to have the same duration as conventional facelifts. The senior author (B.A.M.) has been performing MACS lifts since 2006 and has not yet seen a patient for secondary face-lifting. To date, the longest in-office follow-up has been 8 years.

SUMMARY

Age-related changes in facial anatomy are best addressed using a multimodal approach. The MACS facelift incorporates the principles of facial rejuvenation using a minimal access approach and the use of looped, purse-string sutures. The effect is similar to a composite flap being elevated underneath the skin without the need for surgical delamination. As such, this technique is a powerful and safe tool to restore midface volume and soft tissue descent. Furthermore, the MACS facelift requires less operative time, allowing for the safe accommodation of other facial or nonfacial procedures. Complications, such as hematomas, are also more readily handled owing to the limited and superficial plane of dissection.

However, the MACS facelift technique is not without its limitations, as previously described.[11,12] Nevertheless, the MACS facelift is an effective technique with high levels of physician and patient satisfaction. In the properly selected patient, excellent facial rejuvenation can be achieved, affording a quicker recovery, reduction in operative time and risk, and the potential for concurrent nonfacial procedures.

SUPPLEMENTARY DATA

Supplementary data related to this article can be found online at https://doi.org/10.1016/j.cps.2019.06.005.

REFERENCES

1. Gamboa GM, de La Torre JI, Vasconez LO. Surgical anatomy of the midface as applied to facial rejuvenation. Ann Plast Surg 2004;52(3):240–5.
2. Pessa JE. An algorithm of facial aging: verification of Lambros's theory by three-dimensional stereolithography, with reference to the pathogenesis of midfacial aging, scleral show, and the lateral suborbital trough deformity. Plast Reconstr Surg 2000;106(2):479–88 [discussion: 489–90].
3. Zoumalan RA, Larrabee WF Jr. Anatomic considerations in the aging face. Facial Plast Surg 2011;27(1):16–22.
4. Beale EW, Rasko Y, Rohrich RJ. A 20-year experience with secondary rhytidectomy: a review of technique, longevity, and outcomes. Plast Reconstr Surg 2013;131(3):625–34.
5. Lambros V. Models of facial aging and implications for treatment. Clin Plast Surg 2008;35(3):319–27 [discussion: 317].
6. Stuzin JM, Baker TJ, Baker TM. Refinements in face lifting: enhanced facial contour using vicryl mesh incorporated into SMAS fixation. Plast Reconstr Surg 2000;105(1):290–301.
7. Tonnard P, Verpaele A, Monstrey S, et al. Minimal access cranial suspension lift: a modified S-lift. Plast Reconstr Surg 2002;109(6):2074–86.
8. Tonnard P, Verpaele A. The MACS-lift short scar rhytidectomy. Aesthet Surg J 2007;27(2):188–98.
9. Tonnard PL, Verpaele A, Gaia S. Optimising results from minimal access cranial suspension lifting (MACS-lift). Aesthetic Plast Surg 2005;29(4):213–20 [discussion: 221].
10. Fogli AL. Skin and platysma muscle anchoring. Aesthetic Plast Surg 2008;32(3):531–41.
11. Buchanan PJ, Mihora DC, Mast BA. Facelift practice evolution: objective implementation of new surgical techniques. Ann Plast Surg 2018;80(6S Suppl 6):S324–7.
12. Mast BA. Advantages and limitations of the MACS lift for facial rejuvenation. Ann Plast Surg 2014;72(6):S139–43.
13. Jewell ML. Facelift: facial rejuvenation with loop sutures–the MACS lift and its derivatives. In: Rubin RJ, Neligan PC, editors. Plastic surgery, Vol. 2. 4th edition. Canada: Elsevier; 2018. p. 153–66.

Facelift in Patients with Massive Weight Loss

Rafael A. Couto, MD[a], Ali H. Charafeddine, MD[b], James E. Zins, MD[a],*

KEYWORDS

- Facelift • Fat transfer • Massive weight loss • Necklift • Platysmaplasty • SMAS

KEY POINTS

- Age, gender, preoperative weight, amount and rapidity of weight loss, and degree of skin inelasticity can impact the grade of facial aging in patients with massive weight loss.
- The probability of a staged or revision procedure should be discussed preoperatively.
- Longer incisions along the posterior and anterior hairline are often necessary to remove the excess skin and avoid hairline step-offs.
- Wide skin undermining is the most critical part of the massive weight loss facelift, as it will optimize skin redraping and enable access to the mobile superficial musculoaponeurotic system.
- Fat grafting of the deep malar compartment is a useful ancillary procedure for the treatment of midface deflation.

INTRODUCTION

In 2013, the American Medical Association classified morbid obesity as a distinct disease entity.[1] Bariatric surgery has become an increasingly common therapy for obese patients, leading in most cases to an improved quality of life.[1–5] Patients who undergo massive weight loss (MWL) through either surgical intervention or diet and exercise alone have a significant reduction of their body fat and weight-related comorbidities.[6–8] This rapid decrease in body mass often leads to skin excess, causing physical and psychosocial morbidity.[9–15] Consequently, patients become displeased with their physical appearance. This may result in patients seeking post-MWL body contouring.[9–15] Because most of the of the body fat loss occurs in the trunk and extremities, this patient population pursues body contouring procedures more commonly than facial rejuvenation surgery. However, patients with MWL can also experience significant cervicofacial changes exacerbating the appearance of true facial age.[16,17]

The facial skin excess and laxity seen in the patient with MWL is analogous to the MWL population presenting for body contouring. The result is a deflated skin/soft tissue envelope with poor contractility.[18–20] Although the resultant laxity affects the skin, superficial musculoaponeurotic system (SMAS), and platysma, the skin excess predominates over the laxity in the SMAS and platysma.[16,21–23]

Body contouring following MWL is well documented in the plastic surgery literature; however, there is a paucity of information addressing cervicofacial aging and rejuvenation in this patient population.[16,17,21–23] Although the facelift approach in the MWL patient population is similar to the general population, this patient group also presents with unique challenges. Therefore, there are several modifications that need to be considered to ensure a successful outcome.

PREOPERATIVE MANAGEMENT

Comprehensive evaluation of the patient with MWL is essential to minimizing complications. Examination should include medical and surgical history, with special attention to the weight loss, including (1) maximum weight/body mass index

Disclosure: The authors have nothing to disclose.
[a] Department of Plastic Surgery, Cleveland Clinic Foundation, 9500 Euclid Avenue, Cleveland, OH 44195, USA;
[b] Center for Plastic & Reconstructive Surgery, 5333 McAuley Drive, Suite 5001, Ypsilanti, MI 48197, USA
* Corresponding author.
E-mail address: zinsj@ccf.org

(BMI), (2) current weight/BMI, (3) total weight loss, (4) ultimate weight loss goal, and (5) type of weight loss.[10] Similar to any MWL body contouring procedure, facelift surgery should be deferred for 6 to 12 months after the patient's weight has stabilized.[23] This time will allow for any residual skin contraction to take place. Performing a facelift procedure on a patient who is currently losing weight can lead to an undercorrected facial rejuvenation, as there is greater risk for recurrence of skin excess and volume deflation.

Although weight loss can reduce some of the medical comorbidities typically encountered in this patient population, often there are remaining health issues that require proper workup. Therefore, collaboration with the patient's primary care physician is recommended. A full metabolic workup to assess the possibility of malnutrition is indicated, as this can lead to wound-healing complications or other adverse events.[10] Iron deficiency is observed in up to 50% of the post–bariatric surgery population, which can lead to iron deficiency anemia.[10] Deficiencies in calcium, zinc, vitamin B-12, fat-soluble vitamins (A,D,E,K), and protein are associated in this patient population.[10] Glycemic levels need to be evaluated, and if not controlled, must be optimized before surgery. Furthermore, a detailed cardiovascular examination should be performed to rule out any cardiac abnormalities.

Approximately 40% of patients with MWL have a diagnosed psychiatric disorder at the time of plastic surgery consultation.[24] Recognizing the psychosocial comorbidities affecting this patient population is crucial for deciding whether to perform the procedure in the first place, as well as setting expectations preoperatively. Individuals taking serotonergic antidepressant and antipsychotic drugs have an increased risk of bleeding; therefore, this should be included in the preoperative discussion.[25] Last, they should be counseled that a revision and/or staged procedures might be necessary to obtain optimal results depending on the degree of skin laxity and excess.[16,23]

A thorough preoperative analysis and accurate delineation of the aesthetic goals are critical for a good result.[26] Preoperatively communicating to the patient the areas of asymmetry avoids potential postoperative misunderstandings. Following a methodical approach to facial analysis is essential. A simple method for a soft tissue cephalometric evaluation is to divide the face into equal thirds along trichion, glabella, subnasale, and menton (**Fig. 1**A).[27] Transversely, the face can be segmentally split into 5 equal portions, the width of each equals the width of one eye.[27] In profile view, the soft tissue pogonion should fall on a tangent

from the upper lip to the lower lip (Riedel line) (**Fig. 1**B).[28] Identifying sagittal and/or vertical microgenia in the lower face is important, given that chin implants and horizontal genioplasties are simple techniques that can enhance jaw definition and improve neck contour of these patients.[27,28] The upper to lower lip ratio should be 1-to-2, with 2 to 3 mm of incisor show at repose and up to a full incisor crown display during smile.[27,28] The bigonial distance is approximately 30% less than the bizygomatic, and the gonial angle should be in line with the lateral canthus.[27] Transverse deficiencies can be addressed by gonial angle implants. In benign masseteric hypertrophy, the bigonial distance is increased.[27] All these treatment options should be presented to the patient, and discussed whether it is preferable to do these procedures concomitantly with the facelift or as a staged procedure.[16]

The characteristic findings in the upper face of the patient with MWL are temporal hollowing and prominence of the lateral orbital rim (**Fig. 2**).[16,23] However, other age-related changes can be found and should be assessed. MWL facelift requires extended incisions and placement of the incision along the hairline; therefore, patients must be evaluated for frontal and temporal recession. The ideal frontal hairline is approximately 6 cm from the brow at the pupil in women and 6 to 7 cm in men. Women with frontal recession (≥7 cm) can benefit from hairline-lowering procedures. A hairline incision can be used to correct brow ptosis. Other age-related findings in the patient with brow ptosis include compensatory forehead rhytids, glabellar and frown lines, and periorbital temporal laugh lines (crow's feet).

Although midface volume deflation, descent of the cheek, and attenuation of the orbital septum submalar hollowness are often found in the facial aging patient, these qualities are especially prominent in the patient with MWL (see **Fig. 2**).[29–33] Furthermore, the significant malar deflation and central face laxity observed in the patient with MWL can intensify the nasolabial folds and cervicofacial creases (**Figs. 3** and **4**).[16,23] Although the eyelids are critical elements of facial rejuvenation,[32] their detailed clinical assessment and sophisticated treatment options are beyond the scope of this article.

The lower third of the face in the patient with MWL is distinguished by heavy jowls, perioral rhytids, and marked marionette lines (see **Figs. 3** and **4**).[16,23] Malar descent and jowling obscure jaw definition and can result in a square or masculinized lower face.[28,33] The corner of the mouth should be roughly in line with the medial limbus of the cornea.[27] Upper lip elongation is a common

A

B

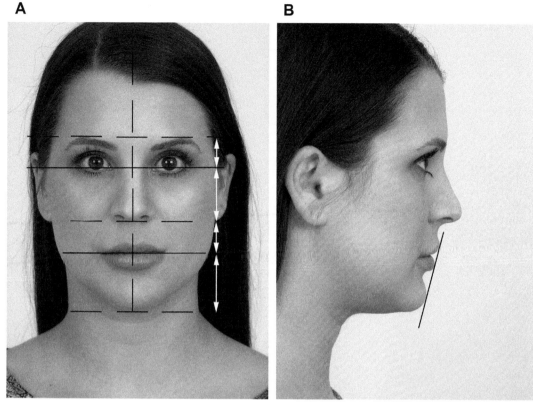

Fig. 1. (*A*) Front view of the face of a 31-year-old woman. The face can be divided into equal thirds along trichion, glabella, and subnasale. Distance from the medial canthus to top of the brow is approximately equal to the distance of alar base to the oral commissure. The distance from the alar base to the oral commissure is approximately half the distance from the oral commissure to the soft tissue menton. (*B*) Profile view of the face and neck of a 31-year old woman. The face can be divided into equal thirds. In the lower third the upper lip to lower lip ratio should be 1:2. To assess the sagittal relations of the upper and lower jaw a tangent from the pogonion (soft tissue menton) to the nasal tip should be roughly touching the lips.

feature of the aging face that can be corrected with lip lift techniques.[28,34] Perioral rhytids also may be present and are best addressed at the time of facelift with chemical or laser resurfacing modalities.[16,23,35]

Last, the MWL neck is often characterized by severe skin excess and platysmal laxity.[16,21–23] Clinically, these present as vertical banding, skin redundancy, and an obtuse cervicomental angle (see **Figs. 3** and **4**; **Fig. 5**).[16,33,36–39] Although subplatysmal fat and anterior digastric fullness are less evident than the excess neck skin and platysmal laxity, they should be assessed intraoperatively.

OPERATIVE TECHNIQUE

Preoperatively, the patient is marked in a seated upright position. Useful landmarks include the extent of planned skin undermining, location of the jowls, and prominent platysmal bands.

Facelifts for patients with MWL are performed under general anesthesia or conscious sedation in an accredited outpatient surgery center or hospital facility. Preoperative antibiotics are administered at least 30 minutes before incision. If there is no history of allergy to cephalosporin antibiotics, the patient receives 2 g of cefazolin. In the case of cephalosporin allergy, 600 mg of clindamycin is administered. If indicated, antibiotics may be re-dosed intraoperatively. Postoperative antibiotics are not prescribed, nor is there strong evidence advocating their necessity. Lower extremity sequential compression devices are applied before induction of anesthesia. Following intubation, the endotracheal tube may be secured to the mandibular premolar with a 26-gauge wire, covered with a sterile stockinette and placed in a "Christmas tree" tube holder. This configuration allows the surgeon to move the tube freely across the field, and access every facial region without risks to the airway.[40] The patient is prepped

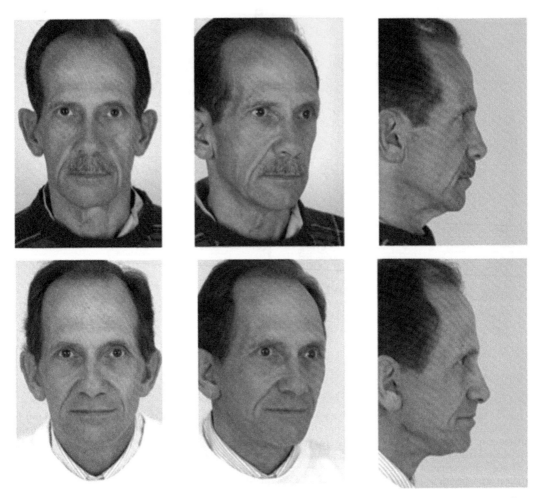

Fig. 2. A 57-year-old man with history of 140-pound weight loss after undergoing gastric bypass surgery. The patient's primary concern was his submalar and temporal hollowing, pronounced nasolabial folds, and marionette lines (*top*). An extended SMAS facelift combined bilateral submalar implants was performed. Note the improved the submalar hollowing after placement of the implants. He is shown 5 months after surgery (*bottom*).

down to the clavicle with betadine, and draped in the usual sterile fashion. If fat grafting is planned, harvesting sites also are prepped and squared off with towels at this time. We prefer to use a local infiltration solution containing 0.5% lidocaine and 1:200,000 epinephrine, which has been suggested to produce sufficient vasoconstriction to obtain an essentially bloodless field.[37,41,42]

Skin Incision Planning

Although planning skin incisions and anticipating skin repositioning are important in all facelift surgery, it is particularly important in this patient population.[16,21–23] The MWL facelift may often require a longer incision along the posterior hairline to enable the removal of excess neck skin and repositioning of the skin flap in a posterior vector, while avoiding a hairline step-off.[16,22,23] For similar reasons, an anterior hairline incision in the temporal region may be preferred.[16,22,23] The neck is accessed anteriorly through a 3.5-cm submental incision that is made approximately 1 cm anterior or posterior to the submental crease, but not in the crease.

Management of Skin Laxity

The main problem that needs to be addressed in a MWL facelift is the skin redundancy that often exceeds the superficial fascial laxity.[16,21–23] Therefore, wide skin undermining is imperative to achieve a successful cervicofacial rejuvenation in this patient population (**Fig. 6**). Subcutaneous undermining is performed with special care to maintain an appropriate layer of fat over the SMAS, especially in the malar and submalar

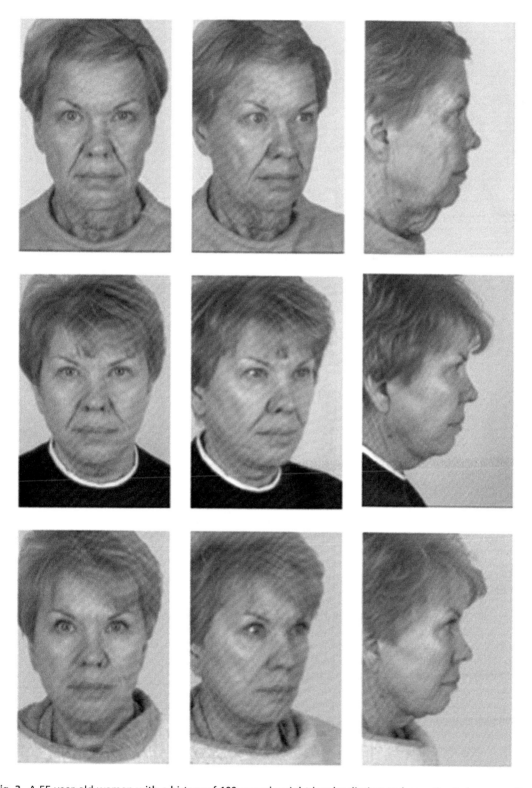

Fig. 3. A 55-year-old woman with a history of 100-pound weight loss by dieting and an estimated preoperative apparent age of 69.4 years old (*top*). She underwent a 2-staged procedure: an extended SMAS facelift combined with an upper eyelid blepharoplasty and platysmaplasty (*middle*), followed by a direct excision of nasolabial fold and CO_2 laser resurfacing 8 months later (*bottom*). Although the patient would benefit from revision on the

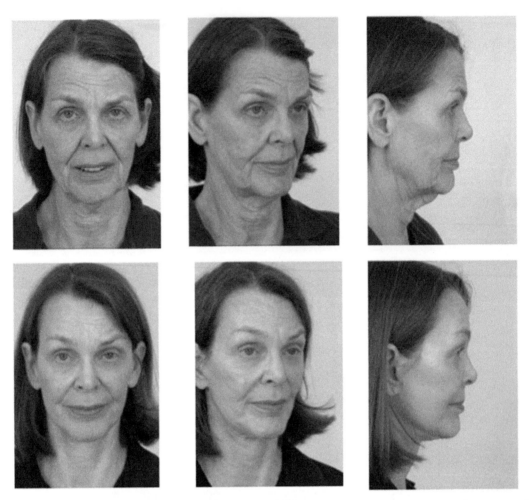

Fig. 4. A 64-year-old woman who lost 108 pounds by dieting with a preoperative apparent age of 65.4 years old (*Top*). The patient underwent an SMAS facelift combined with an endoscopic brow lift and platysmaplasty was performed. Five months later, direct nasolabial fold excision, perioral phenol-croton oil peel, and CO_2 laser resurfacing as revision procedure. Twelve months after the rhytidectomy, her postoperative apparent age was 60 years old and apparent age reduction was 6.4 years (*bottom*). (*From* Couto RA, Waltzman JT, Tadisina KK, et al. Objective assessment of facial rejuvenation after massive weight loss. Aesthetic Plast Surg. 2015;39(6):852; with permission.)

regions, and in addition, leaving fat on the SMAS adds surprising strength to this layer.[43] In the temporal region, the extent of skin undermining extends to the orbicularis oculi muscle, whereas in the cheek area the dissection stops at the start of zygomaticus major muscle. Skin flap dissection is gradually continued anteriorly to release the mandibular septum and ligament. Releasing these structures will provide easier access to the submental region, and decrease tethering around the jawline. Finally, the neck is dissected in a supra-platysmal plane and taken across the midline, submental region to join the facial skin flaps (see **Fig. 6**).

Management of the Superficial Musculoaponeurotic System

Although the senior author (JEZ) uses the SMAS technique (ie, extended SMAS, SMAS plication,

cervical region, the patient was content with the results achieved and did not desire additional procedures. Sixteen months after the facelift, her postoperative apparent age was 60.9 years old; therefore, apparent age reduction was 9.5 years (*bottom*). (*Modified from* Couto RA, Waltzman JT, Tadisina KK, et al. Objective assessment of facial rejuvenation after massive weight loss. Aesthetic Plast Surg. 2015;39(6):851; with permission.)

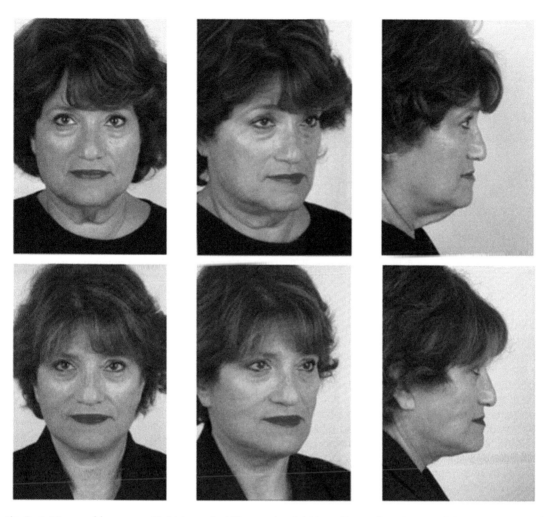

Fig. 5. A 57-year-old woman with history of a 100-pound weight loss after undergoing gastric bypass surgery and a preoperative apparent age of 59.6 years old (*top*). She underwent an extended SMAS facelift and transconjunctival lower lid blepharoplasty. On her 8-month follow-up photograph, her estimated postoperative apparent age was 56.8 years old; thus, apparent age reduction was 2.9 years (*bottom*). (*From* Couto RA, Waltzman JT, Tadisina KK, et al. Objective assessment of facial rejuvenation after massive weight loss. Aesthetic Plast Surg. 2015;39(6):853; with permission.)

SMASectomy) that best fits the patient's anatomy, the extended SMAS dissection is the most common approach used during an MWL facelift.[16]

Once wide skin undermining has been completed, attention is turned to the SMAS. The upper extent of the SMAS flap is designed at the lower border of zygomatic arch.[44,45] Once the middle third of the zygomatic arch is passed, there is no risk of facial nerve injury. Thus, the upper edge of the SMAS flap is directed cranially toward the lateral canthus for 2 cm, and then caudally toward the nasolabial fold for 2 cm. This design enables the surgeon to include the bulk of the malar fat pad into the SMAS flap. The flap is raised from the pre-auricular area parallel to the ear and

extends 2 cm behind the gonial angle into the posterior border of the platysma muscle. The sub-SMAS dissection leaves fat over the masseteric fascia, and ensuring that the facial nerve branches are protected. Release of the zygomatic and masseteric ligaments will lead to the visualization of the zygomaticus major muscle. Dissecting medial to the zygomaticus major muscle will release any remaining zygomatic ligaments, whereas caudal dissection will divide the upper masseteric ligaments.[43] Using blunt spreading motion, dissection proceeds superficial to the Zygomaticus Major (ZM) muscle toward the nasolabial crease. Although this maneuver will maximize fat translation, it should be performed with caution in

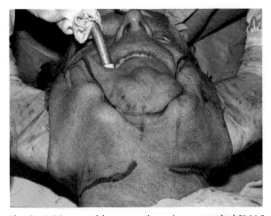

Fig. 6. A 66-year-old man undergoing extended SMAS facelift and upper lid blepharoplasty. Wide skin undermining is the most critical part of the MWL facelift. It will facilitate the resection of the excess skin and the posterior/horizontal vector repositioning of the neck skin flaps.

the MWL facelift, as the aforementioned skin flap dissection may extend beyond the medial limit of the SMAS flap, and thus risk transection of the SMAS while undermining it medially. The SMAS flap is then transposed in a superior-lateral vector, parallel to the ZM. The exact fixation point in the deep temporal fascia is determined by observing the cervicofacial effect produced while mobilizing the SMAS flap.[44,45] Following fixation, the posterior edge of the SMAS flap is incised vertically to create an inferiorly based tongue of SMAS. This is transposed posteriorly and anchored to the mastoid fascia and periosteum; thus, tightening the lower mandibular border and neck.[43,45] Please refer to the article by Ali H. Charafeddine and James E. Zins's article, "The Extended SMAS", elsewhere in this issue, for further description and figures of the extended SMAS technique.

Management of the Neck

The soft tissue of the neck typically has a great capacity to contract and adjusts to the contour of the neck; however, in the MWL population this may not be the case. Wide undermining of the neck skin is crucial to address the significant neck skin redundancy and laxity present in this patient population and allows appropriate tensionless repositioning of the neck skin. An anterior approach neck rejuvenation is almost universal in the MWL facelift.[16,22,23]

The neck is accessed through a submental incision that is placed approximately 1 cm anterior or posterior to the submental crease and is approximately 3 cm in length. Anteriorly, the supraplatysmal fat, if present, is directly excised, and then the platysma is opened medially and undermined laterally up to the level of the anterior digastric muscle. Conservative contouring of the subplatysmal fat can be performed at this time; defatting should be limited to the level of the anterior digastric muscle. The platysma laxity is most evident medially; therefore, the platysma is medially plicated using the platysmaplasty of choice.[36] This technique consists of 2-layer running closure of the medial platysmal edges with a second layer imbrication that is lateral to the first platysmal line of repair. The suture is started in the submental region, extended down to the thyroid cartilage, and then is continued up to the chin and halfway down again.[36] Our suture of choice is usually a long-lasting absorbable suture, such as Polydioxanone, or a permanent stitch like Mersiline (Ethicon, Somerville, NJ). For a detailed description of the anterior approach necklift, please refer to the article by Charafeddine and colleagues' article "Neck Rejuvenation: Anatomy and Technique", elsewhere in this issue.

Management of Volume Deflation

Facial volume deflation in patient with MWL is best treated by a combination of facelift and fat injections. In the MWL population, volume recession may result in (1) temporal hollowing and prominent lateral orbital rims, (2) submalar hollowing and deep nasolabial folds, and (3) buccal hollows.[16,17,22,23] Fat grafting of the temporal and deep periorbital region can help correct any temporal concavity deformity or orbital rim protrusion.[46] Furthermore, volumizing the deep malar and nasolabial fat compartments will treat the midface region, and will soften the nasolabial crease (see **Figs. 5** and **6**). Filling the oral commissure will address the buccal hollowing.[46] Compared with the non-MWL, the patient with MWL commonly requires a greater amount fat transfer to achieve the desired correction.

An underused alternative to fat transfer for the submalar hollows is to use a submalar implant.[16,47] Not only it can provide effective and consistent results, but also it can be readily placed at the time of the facelift operation (see **Fig. 2**).[16,47] Please refer to the articles by Rod J. Rohrich and colleagues' article, "The Lift-and-Fill Facelift: SMAS-Manipulation with Fat Compartment Augmentation" and Ziyad S. Hammoudeh and W. Grant Stevens's article, "Nonsurgical Adjuncts Following Facelift to Achieve Optimal Aesthetic Outcomes: "Icing on the Cake"", elsewhere in this issue, for a detail description of the facial fat compartments and the relevant anatomy for facial volumization.

Ancillary Procedures

The MWL facelift can be complemented with adjunct procedures; however, their benefits need to be weighed against the risk of extending the time the patient is under general anesthesia.[48] Although not limited to, the most common ancillary procedures in addition to lipofilling include (1) laser/chemical resurfacing, (2) browlift, (3) upper/lower blepharoplasty, (4) ear lobe reduction, and (5) lip lift (see **Fig. 5**; **Fig. 7**).[16,23] Resurfacing the face at the time of the facelift has been advocated by several investigators and has been shown to be safe in the general population.[49] However, concomitant skin resurfacing during an MWL face-lift should be limited to areas that were not undermined. The poor skin quality and extensive skin undermining required in facelifts of patients with MWL may make the skin flaps more susceptible to wound-healing complications. Conversely, a staged resurfacing allows for treatment of the entire face with less concern for compromising the skin flaps.[23]

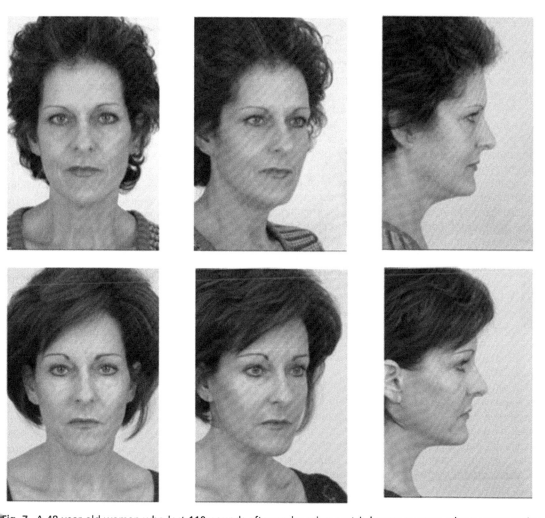

Fig. 7. A 48-year-old woman who lost 110 pounds after undergoing gastric bypass surgery, whose preoperative apparent age was 52.7 years old. Note how the MWL facial changes are less evident in this individual compared with other patients. The variability of excess skin and volume deflation is profound. The greater skin elasticity in younger patients may afford greater tolerance of facial aging in the setting of MWL (*top*). The patient underwent an extended SMAS face lift combined with endoscopic browlift, periocular laser resurfacing, and fat injections to the cheeks, nasolabial folds, infraorbital rims, and lips. A revision of endoscopic brow lift was performed 10 months later. She is shown 32 months after the rhytidectomy; her postoperative apparent age was 49.3 years old and apparent age reduction was 4.4 years (*bottom*). (*From* Couto RA, Waltzman JT, Tadisina KK, et al. Objective assessment of facial rejuvenation after massive weight loss. Aesthetic Plast Surg. 2015;39(6):854; with permission.)

DISCUSSION

The facial changes of patients with MWL mimic the age-related findings observed in the non-MWL population. There appears to be diminished subcutaneous fat and enhanced loss of skin elasticity. Therefore, exaggerated facial aging occurs, and patients with MWL appear older than their actual age.[16,17] Although the non-MWL population goes through the expected facial aging findings (eg, SMAS laxity, retaining ligament attenuation, volume deflation, loss of skin elasticity), the patient with MWL goes through both (1) aging associated skin/soft tissue changes; and (2) skin/soft tissue alterations associated with the process of expansion and rapid deflation. These 2 acting independent factors may explain why patients with MWL look significantly older than their non-MWL counterparts: the natural aging process plus negative changes from MWL itself. Valente and colleagues[17] demonstrated that men older than 40 years, with a preoperative BMI of more than 40 kg/m^2, preoperative weight more than 127 kg, and percentage of excess weight lost greater than 75% had a greater perceived facial aging. Unfortunately, the investigators were unable to determine which factor correlated most strongly with changes in facial aging. Nonetheless, a fact is that skin laxity is the main contributor of the facial deformity seen in the patient with MWL, and all these factors can directly and/or indirectly impact the quality and elastic properties of the skin.[49–51] In our experience, we feel that age may be the most important factor influencing (1) the degree of facial deformity, (2) the apparent facial aging appearance, and (3) the facelift longevity in the MWL population. The greater skin elasticity in younger patients may correspond to improved tolerance of facial aging in the setting of MWL (see **Fig. 7**).[17,22]

Facelift after MWL enhances cervicofacial appearance[16,21,22] and reduces apparent facial aging (see **Figs. 3–7**).[16] In a recent study, we used the concept of "apparent age" as a mean to objectify the results of MWL facelift surgery.[16,52] Although our patients with MWL appeared 5.1 years older than their actual age, our findings of a 6 years reduction in apparent age were similar both in the MWL and non-MWL group.[16] Both volume deflation and skin redundancy are the overriding factors in their facial aging.[16,21,22] Therefore, wide skin undermining and volume repletion are the most crucial parts of this operation. Narasimhan and colleagues[22] showed that an average of 3.0 cm and 1.5 cm of skin is resected in the MWL and non-MWL facelift, respectively. A greater amount of skin resection requires longer incisions to adequately re-drape the skin flaps. Therefore, incisions often need to be placed along the posterior and temporal hairline to avoid hairline step-offs.[16,21–23] The senior author repositions the facial and neck skin in a vertical-oblique and posterior vector, respectively.[16] However, others have suggested to accommodate the facial skin in a vertical[21,22] direction and to reposition the neck skin in a superior[21] or postero-superior[22] vector.

A wide variety of face and neck rejuvenation techniques (eg, sub-SMAS dissection, SMAS plication, and SMASectomy) have been described.[43,53–56] Although surgeons often adopt a particular technique over all others, the literature has not shown a clear superiority among facelift techniques when addressing facial aging in patients in general.[57–62] The MWL facelift skin undermining generally needs to be more extensive, especially in the neck, and should be accompanied by a medial platysmaplasty. The senior author uses the SMAS technique (eg, SMAS plication, sub-SMAS dissection, SMASectomy) that benefits the patient's facial anatomy the most; however, the extended SMAS is the approach most commonly used for MWL facelifts.[16]

The bilamellar dissection involved in the extended SMAS-lift, enables the surgeon to independently reposition the SMAS and the skin in different vectors. The argument for a unilamellar approach (eg, composite facelift) is that blood supply is maximized and combines the benefits of resistance to suture tearing and less stress relaxation.[63] Although we prefer to reposition the SMAS in a vertical direction,[16] other investigators accommodate the SMAS either in an oblique or a vertical position, depending of the patient's facial anatomy.[22] The ultimate goal is to use the SMAS as a mean to reposition the facial fat compartments, restore midface volume, and redefine the jawline. Although comparable vectors can be achieved with the other SMAS techniques, in the extended SMAS, theoretically, a greater level of SMAS excursion can be accomplished. In a sub-SMAS dissection, the SMAS is freed off the parotidomasseteric fascia, and released from the zygomatic and upper masseteric ligaments before changing to the subcutaneous plane distal to the ZM, thus allowing an effective SMAS reposition.[43,64] Because the SMAS is in continuity with the platysma, a structure with minimal osseous attachment to the mandible,[43] the superior-posterior SMAS repositioning achieved with a sub-SMAS dissection should translate into a greater platysma tightening. Therefore, the SMAS is not only acting as a vehicle to passively reposition fat back to the face, but also an instrument to restore neck contour and jawline definition.[43]

There is an inherent risk of increased complications when opening the neck during a facelift; however, we believe that the benefits of performing an anterior necklift approach outweigh their risks, especially in the MWL population. Their skin excess is mostly noted in the neck region; the skin does not contract and/or adjust to neck contour as observed in the non-MWL population. Consequently, the skin pulls away from the neck structures, causing platysmal banding and an obtuse cervicomental angle in addition to skin redundancy.[16,21–23] To address the neck skin laxity and adequately re-drape it, wide subcutaneous dissection must be performed. The most appropriate way to accomplish this is through the facelift and submental incisions.[16,22,23]

Platysmal laxity is greatest medially; therefore, a midline platysmaplasty through a submental incision is the best approach.[36] Other investigators also recognize the important role that a midline platysmaplasty plays in the correction of the MWL neck.[21,22] If lateral platysma laxity needs to be addressed, a lateral platysmal window technique[65] has been suggested to better define the jawline.[22] A variety of spanning sutures have been described for improving the jawline and mandibular angle.[37,66–68] However, this is particularly ineffective in the MWL population. The long-term efficacy of suspension sutures in correcting deformities deep to the platysma is questioned.[39,69,70] In addition, untoward effects of these techniques are a real risk.

In spite of all the previously described precautions and modifications, the large skin excess and marked skin laxity present in the MWL population may still lead to early skin creep under correction in both the neck and nasolabial folds. Therefore, early recurrence and the probability of a secondary is likely. In our study, revision procedures were more frequent in the MWL facelift (42.8%) compared with the non-MWL patient (9.1%).[16] The revision procedures included direct nasolabial fold excision, fat grafting, laser resurfacing, and perioral chemical peeling. Rawlani and Mustoe[63] addressed these challenges by staging the facelift in a similar patient population. They found a benefit to using a secondary procedure involving delayed flaps and reduced stress relaxation and creep, thus allowing a greater tension to be applied on skin closure.[63] During a staged facelift, the surgeon maintains better control of the final surgical result and the patient's expectations. Facelift revision surgery not only enables for further correction resulting from enhanced skin creep, but also offers the surgeon and patient an opportunity to address additional areas of concern through ancillary procedures, including repeat fat grafting, skin resurfacing, and a variety of forehead procedures (see **Figs. 3**, **4**, and **7**). One procedure unique to the MWL population deserves to be mentioned. Direct nasolabial fold excision can occasionally be used to great benefit by excising skin where laxity is greatest.[16,71–75] This procedure can have a decided beneficial effect (see **Figs. 3** and **4**).

SUMMARY

Patients with MWL exhibit accelerated facial aging, often appearing older than their stated age. Facelift can enhance the cervicofacial appearance, and significantly reduce the patient's perceived age. The MWL facelift presents unique challenges to achieving short-term or long-term correction. Therefore, a discussion about patient expectation and the likelihood of revision or staged procedure is imperative to ensure successful outcomes.

REFERENCES

1. Ortiz SE, Kawachi I, Boyce AM. The medicalization of obesity, bariatric surgery, and population health. Health 2017;21(5):498–518.
2. Trus TL, Pope GD, Finlayson SR. National trends in utilization and outcomes of bariatric surgery. Surg Endosc 2005;19(5):616–20.
3. Rosenberg PH, Henderson KE, Grilo CM. Psychiatric disorder comorbidity and association with eating disorders in bariatric surgery patients: a cross-sectional study using structured interview-based diagnosis. J Clin Psychiatry 2006;67(7):1080–5.
4. Kalarchian MA, Marcus MD, Levine MD, et al. Psychiatric disorders among bariatric surgery candidates: relationship to obesity and functional health status. Am J Psychiatry 2007;164(2):328–34, 374.
5. Khan S, Rock K, Baskara A, et al. Trends in bariatric surgery from 2008 to 2012. Am J Surg 2016;211:1041–6.
6. Poyatos JV, Balibrea JM, Sales BO, et al. Post-bariatric surgery body contouring treatment in the public health system: cost study and perception by patients. Plast Reconstr Surg 2014;134(3):448–54.
7. Salminen P, Helmiö M, Ovaska J, et al. Effect of laparoscopic sleeve gastrectomy versus laparoscopic Roux-en-Y gastric bypass on weight loss at 5 years among patients with morbid obesity: the SLEEVEPASS randomized clinical trial. JAMA 2018;319:241–54.
8. Peterli R, Wölnerhanssen BK, Peters T, et al. Effect of laparoscopic sleeve gastrectomy versus laparoscopic Roux-en-Y gastric bypass on weight loss in

patients with morbid obesity: the SM-BOSS random-ized clinical trial. JAMA 2018;319:255–65.

9. Taylor J, Shermak M. Body contouring following massive weight loss. Obes Surg 2004;14:1080–5.

10. Bossert RP, Rubin JP. Evaluation of the weight loss patient presenting for plastic surgery consultation. Plast Reconstr Surg 2012;130:1361–9.

11. Friedman T, O'Brien CD, Michaels J, et al. Fleur-de-Lis abdominoplasty: a safe alternative to traditional abdominoplasty for the massive weight loss patient. Plast Reconstr Surg 2010;125:1525–35.

12. Kitzinger HB, Abayev S, Pittermann A, et al. The prevalence of body contouring surgery after gastric bypass surgery. Obes Surg 2012;22:8–12.

13. Mitchell JE, Crosby RD, Ertelt TW, et al. The desire for body contouring surgery after bariatric surgery. Obes Surg 2008;18:1308–12.

14. Sioka E, Tzovaras G, Katsogridaki G, et al. Desire for body contouring surgery after laparoscopic sleeve gastrectomy. Aesthetic Plast Surg 2015;39:978–84.

15. Steffen KJ, Sarwer DB, Thompson JK, et al. Predictors of satisfaction with excess skin and desire for body contouring after bariatric surgery. Surg Obes Relat Dis 2012;8:92–7.

16. Couto RA, Waltzman JT, Tadisina KK, et al. Objective assessment of facial rejuvenation after massive weight loss. Aesthetic Plast Surg 2015; 39:847–55.

17. Valente DS, da Silva JB, Mottin CC, et al. Influence of massive weight loss on the perception of facial age: the face age perception cohort. Plast Reconstr Surg 2018;142(4):481e–7e.

18. Aly AS, Cram AE, Heddens C. Truncal body contouring surgery in the massive weight loss patient. Clin Plast Surg 2004;31:611–24.

19. Aly AS, Al- Zahrani, Cram AE. Lower bodylifts. In: Neligan PC, Warren R, editors. Plastic surgery: volume two: aesthetic. 3rd edition. Oxford (United Kingdom): Elsevier; 2013. p. 568–98.

20. Rubin JP, Nguyen V, Schwentker A. Perioperative management of the post-gastric bypass patient presenting for body contouring surgery. Clin Plast Surg 2006;31:601–10.

21. Sclafani AP. Restoration of the jawline and neck after bariatric surgery. Facial Plast Surg 2005;21(1): 28–32.

22. Narasimhan K, Ramanadham S, Rohrich RJ. Face-lifting in the massive weight loss patient: modifications of our technique for this population. Plast Reconstr Surg 2015;135(2):397–405.

23. Waltzman JT, Zins JE, Couto RA. Face and neck lifting after weight loss. Clin Plast Surg 2019;46: 105–14.

24. Mitchell JE, Selzer FZ, Kalarchian MA. Psychopathology before surgery in the longitudinal assessment of bariatric surgery-3(LABS-3) psychosocial study. Surg Obes Relat Dis 2012;8:533.

25. Verdel BM, Souverein PC, Meenks SD, et al. Use of serotonergic drugs and the risk of bleeding. Clin Phamacol Ther 2011;89(1):89–96.

26. Stuzin JM. Restoring facial shape in face lifting: the role of skeletal support in facial analysis and mid-face soft-tissue repositioning. Plast Reconstr Surg 2007;119(1):362–78.

27. Reyneke JP. Systematic patient evaluation. In: Khoury F, Antoun H, Hadi M, editors. Essentials of orthognathic surgery. 1st edition. Berlin: Quintessence Publishing Co, Inc; 2003. p. 13–68.

28. Fardo D, Zins JE, Nahai F. Facelift (lower face): current technique. In: Mathes S, editor. Plastic surgery. 2nd edition. Atlanta (GA): Elsevier; 2006. p. 275–96.

29. Kpodzo DS, Nahai F, McCord CD. Malar mounds and festoons: review of current management. Aesthet Surg J 2014;34:235–48.

30. Stutman RL, Codner MA. Tear trough deformity: review of anatomy and treatment options. Aesthet Surg J 2012;32:426–40.

31. Lambros V. Cosmetic observations on periorbital and midface aging. Plast Reconstr Surg 2007;120: 1367–77.

32. Hashem AM, Couto RA, Waltzman JT, et al. Evidence-based medicine: a graded approach to lower lid blepharoplasty. Plast Reconstr Surg 2017;139: 139e–50e.

33. Knize DM. Limited incision submental lipectomy and platysmaplasty. Plast Reconstr Surg 1998;101: 473–81.

34. Ramaut L, Tonnard P, Verpaele A, et al. Aging of the upper lip: Part I: a retrospective analysis of metric changes in soft tissue on magnetic resonance imaging. Plast Reconstr Surg 2019;143(2):440–6.

35. Ozturck CE, Huettner F, Ozturck, et al. Outcomes assessment of combination face lift and perioral phenol-croton oil peel. Plast Reconstr Surg 2013; 132(5):743e–58e.

36. Feldman JJ. Corset platysmaplasty. Plast Reconstr Surg 1990;85:333–43.

37. Feldman JJ. Neck lift my way. Plast Reconstr Surg 2014;134:1173–83.

38. Zins JE, Fardo D. The "Anterior-Only" approach to neck rejuvenation: an alternative to face lift surgery. Plast Reconstr Surg 2005;115:1761–8.

39. Zins JE, Menon N. Anterior approach to neck rejuvenation. Aesthet Surg J 2010;30:477–84.

40. Dobryansky M, Morrison CM, Zins JE. Patient draping and endotracheal tube positioning during facelift surgery. Ann Plast Surg 2009;63(1):9–10.

41. Swanson E. Evaluation of face lift skin perfusion and epinephrine effect using laser fluorescence imaging. Plast Reconstr Surg Glob Open 2015;3(8):e484.

42. Jones BM, Grover R. Avoiding hematoma in cervicofacial rhytidectomy: a personal 8-year quest. Reviewing 910 patients. Plast Reconstr Surg 2004; 113:381–7, 390.

43. Stuzin JM, Baker TJ, Gordon HL, et al. Extended SMAS dissection as an approach to midface rejuvenation. Clin Plast Surg 1995;22(2):295–311.

44. Stuzin JM, Baker TJ, Baker TM. Refinements in face lifting: enhanced facial contour using vicryl mesh incorporated into SMAS fixation. Plast Reconstr Surg 2000;105(1):290–301.

45. Stuzin JM. MOC-PSSM CME article: face lifting. Plast Reconstr Surg 2008;121(1 Suppl):1–19.

46. Lamb JP, Surek CC. The temple and the brow. In: Lamb J, Surek C, editors. Facial volumization: an anatomic approach. 1st edition. New York: Thieme; 2018. p. 59–61.

47. Delaney S, Kridel R. Enhancing facelift with simultaneous submalar implant augmentation. Aesthet Surg J 2019;39(4):351–62.

48. Cheng H, Clymer JW, Chen BP, et al. Prolonged operative duration is associated with complications: a systematic review and meta-analysis. J Surg Res 2018;229:134–44.

49. Koch BB, Perkins SW. Simultaneous rhytidectomy and full-face carbon dioxide laser resurfacing. Arch Facial Plast Surg 2002;4:227–32.

50. Orpheu SC, Coltro PS, Scopel GP, et al. Collagen and elastic content of abdominal skin after surgical weight loss. Obes Surg 2010;20:480–96.

51. Luebberding S, Krueger N, Kerscher M. Mechanical properties of human skin in vivo: a comparative evaluation in 300 men and women. Skin Res Technol 2014;20(2):127–35.

52. Sami K, Elshahat A, Moussa M, et al. Image analyzer study of the skin in patients with morbid obesity and massive weight loss. Eplasty 2015;23:15e4.

53. Swanson E. Objective assessment of change in apparent age after facial rejuvenation surgery. J Plast Reconstr Aesthet Surg 2011;64(9):1124–31.

54. Tonnard P, Verpaele A, Monstrey S, et al. Minimal access cranial suspension lift: a modified S-lift. Plast Reconstr Surg 2002;109(6):2074–86.

55. Baker DC. Lateral SMASectomy. Plast Reconstr Surg 1997;100(2):509–13.

56. Hamra ST. Building the composite face lift: a personal odyssey. Plast Reconstr Surg 2016;138(1):85–96.

57. Marten TJ. High SMAS facelift: combined single flap lifting of the jawline, cheek, and midface. Clin Plast Surg 2008;35(4):569–603.

58. Burke JP. Should the subcutaneous tissue be plicated in a face lift? Plast Reconstr Surg 1974;54(1):1–4.

59. Rees TD, Aston SJ. A clinical evaluation of the results of submusculo-aponeurotic dissection and fixation in face lifts. Plast Reconstr Surg 1977;59(12):851–9.

60. Smith RC, Karolow WW, Papsidero MJ, et al. Comparison of SMAS plication with SMAS imbrication in face lifting. Laryngoscope 1982;92:901–11.

61. Prado A, Andrades P, Danilla S, et al. A clinical retrospective study comparing two short-scar face lifts: minimal access cranial suspension versus lateral SMASectomy. Plast Recosntr Surg 2006;117(5):1413–25.

62. Antell DE, Orseck MJ. A comparison of face lift techniques in eight consecutive sets of identical twins. Plast Reconstr Surg 2007;120(6):1667–73.

63. Alpert BS, Baker DC, Hamra ST, et al. Identical twin face lifts with different techniques: a 10 year follow up. Plast Reconstr Surg 2009;123(3):1025–33.

64. Rawlani V, Mustoe TA. The staged face lift: addressing the biomechanical limitations of the primary rhytidectomy. Plast Reconstr Surg 2012,130(6):1305–14.

65. Alghoul M, Bitik O, McBride J, et al. Relationship of the zygomatic facial nerve to the retaining ligaments of the face: the Sub-SMAS danger zone. Plast Reconstr Surg 2013;131:245e–52e.

66. Cruz RS, O'Reilly EB, Rohrich RJ. The platysma window: an anatomically safe, efficient, and easily reproducible approach to neck contour in the facelift. Plast Reconstr Surg 2012;129(5):1169–72.

67. Guerrerosantos J. Surgical correction of the fatty fallen neck. Ann Plast Surg 1979;2:389–96.

68. Giampapa VC, Di Bernardo BE. Neck recontouring with suture suspension and liposuction: an alternative for the early rhytidectomy candidate. Aesthetic Plast Surg 1995;19:217–23.

69. Ramirez OM. Advanced considerations determining procedure selection in cervicoplasty. Part two: surgery. Clin Plast Surg 2008;35:691–709.

70. Nahai F. Reconsidering neck suspension sutures. Aesthet Surg J 2004;24:365–7.

71. Zins JE, Waltzman JT, Couto RA. Neck rejuvenation. In: Neligan PC, Rubin P, editors. Plastic surgery: volume two: aesthetic surgery. 4th edition. London: Elsevier; 2018. p. 370–89.

72. Guyuron B, Michelow B. The nasolabial fold: a challenge, a solution. Plast Reconstr Surg 1994;93(3):522–9.

73. Guyuron B. The armamentarium to the recalcitrant nasolabial fold. Clin Plast Surg 1995;22:253.

74. Rudkin G, Miller TA. Aging nasolabial fold and treatment by direct excision. Plast Reconstr Surg 1999;104(5):1502–5.

75. Sen C, Cek DI, Reis M. Direct skin excision fat reshaping and repositioning for correction of prominent nasolabial fold. Aesthetic Plast Surg 2004;28(5):307–11.

Neck Rejuvenation
Anatomy and Technique

Ali H. Charafeddine, MD[a], Rafael A. Couto, MD[b], James E. Zins, MD[c],*

KEYWORDS

• Facelift • Necklift • Rhytidectomy • Platysma window • Corset platysmaplasty

KEY POINTS

- A necklift can be performed as part of the facelift operation or as an independent operation.
- There are 2 general schools of thought in neck rejuvenation: one that approaches the neck through an anterior approach with a submental incision and one that accesses the neck through a posterior approach.
- Understanding the anatomy of the platysma bands and the relation of the platysma to the superficial musculoaponeurotic system is key in performing a successful necklift.
- The key anatomic structures that need to be addressed in every neck rejuvenation procedure include platysma bands, supraplatysma fat, subplatysma fat, anterior digastric muscles, and submandibular glands. A thorough understanding of this anatomy is key to a successful outcome.

 Video content accompanies this article at http://www.plasticsurgery.theclinics.com.

INTRODUCTION

Successful surgical treatment of the aging neck involves manipulation of multiple structures that contribute to the aging process, which can be achieved by studying the aesthetic needs of every patient separately and designing an operative strategy that suits the individual patient.

When planning a neck lift operation, whether isolated or in combination with a facelift, the surgeon must make several decisions. Should an anterior (submental) or posterior (lateral) approach be used? Should the subplatysma layer be addressed? If the subplatysma space is explored, should the anterior belly of the digastrics be reduced? How should the ptotic submandibular glands be treated? If the subplatysma plane has been altered, the platysma must be dealt with. Platysma-modifying techniques include midline plication, partial or complete horizontal transection, and most recently lateral skin displacement.[1]

In this article, the authors provide a detailed review of the important anatomic pearls relevant to the necklift. The technical aspects of the operation and the different platysma-altering techniques are also reviewed.

ANATOMY
Platysma

The platysma is a broad muscle and originates at the deltopectoral fascia and transitions cephalad across the mandibular border as a component of the superficial musculoaponeurotic system (SMAS) (**Fig. 1**). The platysma inserts into the modiolus and acts as a depressor of the lower lip.[2] It is innervated by the cervical branch of the facial nerve. The marginal mandibular nerve (MMN)

Disclosures: The authors have nothing to disclose.
[a] Center for Plastic & Reconstructive Surgery, 5333 McAuley Drive, Suite 5001, Ypsilanti, MI 48197, USA; [b] Cleveland Clinic Foundation, 9500 Euclid Avenue, A60, Cleveland, OH 44195, USA; [c] Department of Plastic Surgery, Cleveland Clinic, 9500 Euclid Avenue, A60, Cleveland, OH 44195, USA
* Corresponding author.
E-mail address: Zinsj@ccf.org

Clin Plastic Surg 46 (2019) 573–586
https://doi.org/10.1016/j.cps.2019.06.004

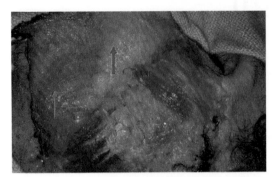

Fig. 1. Cadaver dissection of the left face. An SMAS-platysma flap has been raised. Blue arrow points to the platysma and the red arrow points to the SMAS.

also acts as a lower lip depressor but also innervates the mentalis muscles, providing the ability to evert the lower lip.

De Castro described 3 patterns of distribution of platysma muscle fibers medially. In the submental area, the platysma forms an inverted V with the tip being either at the chin, just below the chin, or at the level of the thyroid cartilage. In the most common variation, Type I (75%), the platysma fibers interlace for just 1 to 2 cm below the chin. In Type II (15%) the fibers interdigitate in the entire submental area down to the thyroid cartilage. In Type III (10%) the platysma muscle fibers are separate in the entire submental region.[2]

The platysma is continuous with the SMAS superiorly, and caudally, its superficial fascia fuses with the pectoralis and deltoid muscles fascia. The superficial cervical fascia covers the platysma muscle. Maintaining the integrity of this fascia is essential to (1) provide an avascular plane of dissection and (2) maintain a robust platysma that can be manipulated and tightened.[3]

Deep Cervical Fascia

The deep investing layer of the deep cervical fascia envelops the submandibular gland and forms its capsule. This anatomy is relevant especially when intracapsular partial submandibular gland resection is performed. Postoperative bleeding in this compartment can lead to serious compromise of the airway.[2] In his series of submandibular gland reductions, Mendelson reports a 1.8% major complication rate requiring a return to the operating room to manage postoperative hematoma. One of those was potentially fatal secondary to airway compromise.[4]

Retaining Ligaments and Filaments

Feldman's description of the retaining ligaments of the neck provides the most accurate anatomic

detail (**Fig. 2**).[5] There are 6 named retaining ligaments in the neck: (1) mastoid-cutaneous ligaments, (2) platysma-auricular/earlobe ligaments (originally described by David Furnas[6]), (3) lateral sternocleidomastoid (SCM)-cutaneous ligaments, (4) submental ligaments, (5) mandibular osteocutaneous ligaments, and (6) platysma-mandibular ligaments (or septum). He also describes 3 filaments in the neck: (1) medial platysma cutaneous filaments, (2) medial SCM filaments, and (3) skin crease platysma filaments.[5] The function of the ligaments and filaments is to hold the cervical skin in place.

The mandibular osteocutaneous ligaments (MOCL) and platysma mandibular ligaments (PML) are often released in face and neck lift surgery. Our cadaver dissections located the MOCL at 56.2 ± 3.1 mm anterior to the gonial angle along the mandibular border and 9.3 ± 1.6 mm superior to it.[7] The same study showed the PML at 48.5 ± 4.4 mm anterior to the gonial angle along the mandibular border and 1.5 ± 0.8 mm superior to it.[7]

The MOCL defines the anterior border of the marionette lines, whereas the PML defines the degree of descent of the jowl. The release of both ligaments is at times often needed for defining the jawline as well as allowing access medially in the submental area. Dissection in this region should be subcutaneous because the MMN lies immediately deep and superior to these structures.[7]

The Marginal Mandibular Nerve

The MMN exits the parotid gland and travels under the parotid-masseteric fascia until it reaches the facial vessels where it passes from under the deep fascia to a sub-SMAS location. It crosses the facial artery at 23.1 mm from the gonial angle and 3.1 mm superior to it (approximately one-fourth of the distance from the gonial angle to

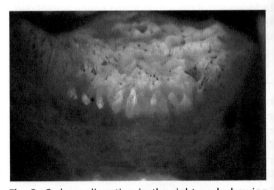

Fig. 2. Cadaver dissection in the right neck showing platysma cutaneous ligaments (*black star*). The skin has been raised and transilluminated.

the pogonion): this is the danger zone for the MMN, the location at which it is most vulnerable to injury and sub-SMAS dissection in this area should proceed with caution. The terminal branches of the MMN are constantly located deep to the SMAS at a mean distance of 9.7 ± 1.2 mm superior to the MOCL.[7]

Although the MMN is never subcutaneous, it can be inadvertently injured even with a planned subcutaneous dissection. This happens when rapid blunt scissor dissection passes under the skin with inadvertent penetration of the platysma. Monopolar cautery in this area can also result in neuropraxia. Loop magnification (2.5x), good illumination, and the use of bipolar cautery limits this occurrence.[7]

Cervical Branch of the Facial Nerve

The cervical branch of the facial nerve exits the inferior parotid gland and immediately changes planes from deep to the parotid-masseteric fascia to a subplatysma plane. It has multiple branches, the lowermost being 4.5 cm below the margin of the mandible.[8] Terzis reports 1 to 3 nerve branches entering the undersurface of the superolateral third of the platysma.[9] In their cadaver dissection, Sinno and Thorne identified only one cervical branch of the facial nerve in all 16 cadavers, with branching occurring at the level of the facial vessels to supply the platysma. The main cervical branch continues anteriorly to the medial edge of the platysma below the thyroid cartilage.[10]

The role of the cervical branch of the facial nerve in the formation of platysma bands has been described by Trévidic and Criollo-Lamilla[11] who followed 25 patients with facial paralysis over a 10-year period and found no platysma bands on the paralyzed side when compared with the healthy side. Recurrent platysma banding is a common and frustrating adverse sequela of necklift surgery. Whether denervation of the platysma will play a critical role is yet to be determined.

The Great Auricular Nerve

The great auricular nerve is the most commonly injured nerve in facelift surgery (**Fig. 3**).[12] The following is a fail-safe method designed to avoid nerve injury: a 30-degree angle is designed with the anterior limb drawn perpendicular to Frankfurt horizontal line extending from the middle of the ear lobule. A second line is drawn 30 degrees posterior to this vertical line. The great auricular nerve will be found within the boundaries of this angle 100% of the time. Practically speaking, when

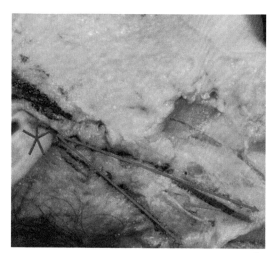

Fig. 3. Cadaver dissection of a right face depicting the danger zone of the great auricular nerve (*blue arrow*). A 30-degree angle is designed (*red arrows*) with the anterior limb bisecting the ear lobule (*blue star*) and perpendicular to Frankfurt horizontal line.

McKinney's point is used to locate the nerve, the nerve is often cut before reaching McKinney's point.

Fat Compartments

The fat compartments of the neck have been extensively studied[13] and divided into 3 regions: (1) superficial or supraplatysma fat (between the platysma and the skin); (2) intermediate or subplatysma fat (between the platysma and the anterior digastric muscles); and deep fat compartment (deep to the anterior digastric and submandibular glands) (**Fig. 4**).

Appropriate fat contouring in both the supraplatysma and intermediate planes can lead to dramatic improvements in necklift results. Conversely, overly aggressive fat removal can lead to complications including contour abnormalities and the cobra deformity.[14]

In the superficial plane a layer of fat approximately 3 mm thick should be left on the neck skin flap to avoid unnatural banding, which is difficult or impossible to correct.

In the intermediate plane, subplatysma defatting should be flush with the anterior belly of the digastrics. Overresection in this area leads to the cobra deformity.[14]

Larson and colleagues[13] measured the weight of the different fat compartments of the neck and concluded that the supraplatysma compartment contains the most amount of fat followed by the intermediate (subplatysma) compartment. The deep fat compartment has the least amount of fat and is not clinically significant.

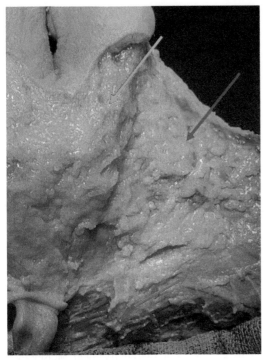

Fig. 4. Cadaver dissection of the right side of the face. During the anterior neck approach, the jowl fat (*green arrow*) is not addressed. The subplatysma fat (*red arrow*) is easily removed. Blue arrow denotes the SCM muscle.

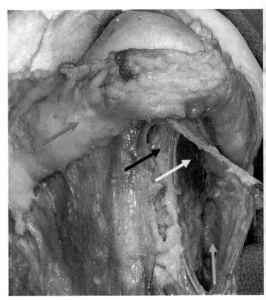

Fig. 5. Cadaver dissection showing relevant anatomy for the neck rejuvenation surgery. Shown are supraplatysma fat (*blue arrow*) lifted, subplatysma fat (*black arrow*), anterior digastric muscle (*yellow arrow*), left submandibular gland (*green arrow*), and raised left platysma (*red arrow*).

PLANNING AND TECHNICAL APPROACH
Anterior Approach to Neck Rejuvenation

The anterior approach (submental) to neck rejuvenation has been reported by multiple investigators.[15–21] Neck skin has a unique ability to contract once separated from the underlying platysma and neck ligaments and filaments.[22,23] Because no skin is removed during an anterior neck approach, the improvement in the degree of the aesthetic result depends on the degree of skin elasticity and not on the cervicomental angle per see. Conversely, the greater the degree of skin laxity, the wider the amount of neck skin undermining is required.

The anterior submental approach allows for manipulation of the following structures: (1) supraplatysma fat, (2) subplatysma fat, (3) anterior digastric muscles (excision, shaving, and plication), (4) submandibular glands, (5) and platysma (tightening procedures).[24,25] All these manipulations done during a facelift surgery can be performed through an anterior approach, except for the indirect tightening resulting from SMAS elevation and reposition[20] (**Fig. 5**).

During the consultation, it is extremely important to explain to the patient that the anterior neck approach will result primarily in improvement in the profile view. Little change will be noted on the front view.[14]

Patients Classification

Patients are classified according to the laxity of their neck skin[14]: Grade I (no laxity), Grade II (mild laxity), Grade III (moderate laxity), and Grade IV (severe laxity). Patients with minimal to no laxity usually can be treated with liposuction alone. However, the surgeon needs to explain to the patient that the diagnosis of subplatysmal fat is hard to do solely on physical examination and the ideal result may require opening the platysma. In general fat necks have subplatysma fat. Therefore, the option of opening the platysma to address this fat gives the surgeon the greatest versatility.

Patients with mild skin laxity (grade II) and an obtuse cervicomental angle are good candidates for the anterior-only neck approach.[14] In those patients, fat in both the supra- and subplatysmal compartments is easily resected. The amount of skin undermining performed is proportional to the degree of skin laxity. A good rule of thumb is the following: the amount of skin undermining should be similar to a face/necklift standard operation. Thus, in patients with mild laxity, skin undermining can be limited, while increasing laxity suggests wider undermining.

In patients with moderate skin laxity (grade III), the skin undermining must be more extensive and extends from the submental midline as far lateral as possible. An additional posterior ear sulcus incision can be added and skin undermined over the SCM through which incision joins the anterior dissection (Video 1).

This operation is generally not suitable for patients with severe skin laxity (grade IV). Those patients are best treated with either a standard face/necklift or in the elderly patient with a direct excision of neck skin and Z-plasty.[26–28]

Skin laxity is not the only factor that comes into play when assessing the neck. Male patients have less impressive results, likely due to less skin contraction after undermining because of the sebaceous nature of the skin. Also, the obese/heavy neck poses a challenge, as it is hard to provide a smooth contour with fat removal only, and these patients often need skin resection.

Ptotic submandibular glands should be noted preoperatively. The anterior approach provides access to the submandibular glands for resection, suspension, or direct platysma plication over the glands. Alternatively, the submandibular glands can be addressed from the lateral approach.[1] Surgeon who perform submandibular gland resection often have a separate consent for this procedure.[24,29]

Surgical technique

Surgical markings are done in the preoperative holding area. The extent of skin undermining is marked while the patient is in the sitting position. Careful examination of the cervicomental angle, the fat compartments, and the submandibular glands are assessed. The operative plan is reviewed with the patient emphasizing what the operation can and cannot do.

This operation can be performed under local anesthesia, local with sedation, or under general anesthesia. The operation is begun by injecting 0.5% lidocaine with 1:200,000 epinephrine, for a total volume of 50 to 60 cc. To this mixture tranexamic acid (TXA) is added at a concentration of 1 mg TXA/1 cc local.

If liposuction is planned, only a stab incision is done in the submental area. The senior author (JEZ) prefers to do fat excision under direct visualization, allowing more accurate fat resection and less trauma to the platysma muscle. If liposuction is performed, care should be taken not to skeletonize the neck, which results in banding or irregularities, problems that are usually hard to correct.

The extent of skin undermining is dictated by the amount of skin laxity (see Video 1). The dissection proceeds on top of the platysma muscle and its investing fascia, leaving all the supraplatysma fat on the skin flap. Preserving the anterior cervical fascia provides strength while performing midline platysmaplasty. Once the appropriate amount of supraplatysma fat is resected, the subplatysma space is explored by opening the platysma in the midline and raising platysma muscle flaps. The lateral extent of the subplatysma dissection is the lateral edge of the anterior belly of the digastric muscles. Subplatysma fat is resected flush with the digastric muscles, with care not to overresect this fat to avoid a submental hollow. The anterior belly of the digastric muscles is assessed for the possible need for resection or plication. The submandibular glands are located just lateral to the anterior belly of the digastric muscles. As dissection proceeds, caudally toward the thyroid cartilage, lymph nodes and bilateral anterior jugular vein branches are routinely encountered. Defatting is performed as far inferior as the thyroid cartilage.

If extended dissection is needed laterally over the SCM fascia, a small postauricular sulcus incision is made bilaterally to complete the dissection laterally. A 7-mm J-VAC drain (Ethicon, Inc., Somerville, New Jersey) is placed to obliterate the dead space. Placement of drains is essential to prevent seromas and to ensure smooth skin redraping.

Postoperatively, the patient is asked to wear a chin strap for 5 days and then for 2 weeks at night only. The drains are removed on postoperative day one.

Anterior Skin Excision and Z-Plasty

Patients who have marked laxity and excess of the neck skin (typically elderly men, aged 60 years and older) are treated with a standard facelift or anterior skin excision and z-plasty (**Fig. 6**, Video 2).[27,30,31] The major drawback in this procedure is a visible scar in the anterior neck. However, this procedure has many benefits including less risk for the elderly population, less recovery time, and excision of skin directly where it is most lax, rather than a standard facelift where the pull is from a more distant site (**Figs. 7** and **8**). This translates into a better and more long-lasting neck correction.[20]

TYPES OF PLATYSMA MANIPULATIONS IN A NECKLIFT OPERATION

Platysma laxity is treated best where laxity is greatest. Platysma manipulations include midline platysma plication, platysma resection with midline closure, and the lateral skin displacement operation. In this section, the authors review the most common platysma manipulations (see **Figs. 6–8**).

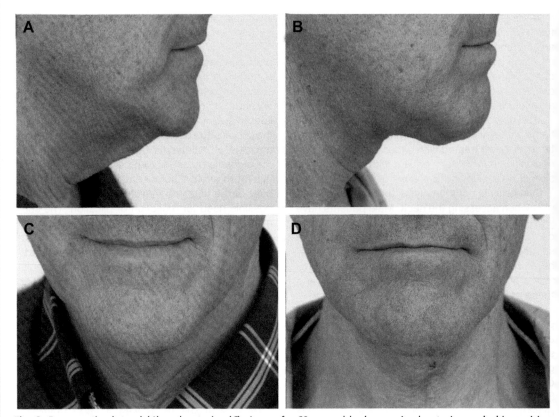

Fig. 6. Preoperative lateral (*A*) and anterior (*C*) views of a 69-year-old who received anterior neck skin excision and z-plasty. Postoperative lateral (*B*) and anterior views (*D*) at a 2-year follow-up are shown.

Corset Platysmaplasty

The corset platysmaplasty was described by Joel Feldman.[5] This technique is performed after the fat compartments have been addressed, in addition to the anterior digastric muscles and the submandibular glands. Leaving the anterior cervical fascia intact on the platysma is one key to the success of this operation. A 3-0 polydioxanone running suture is started anteriorly, with the sutures imbricating the platysma medially and running toward the thyroid cartilage. Once the thyroid cartilage is reached, a second row of imbricating sutures is performed outside the first suture line further tightening the platysma, back to the initial starting point. This can be carried down again. Care should be taken not to tear the platysma during the formation of the corset. Critics

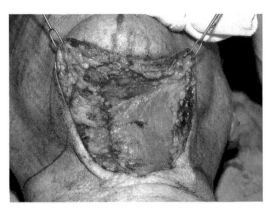

Fig. 7. Intraoperative view of pants-over-vest platysmaplasty from the patient in **Fig. 6**.

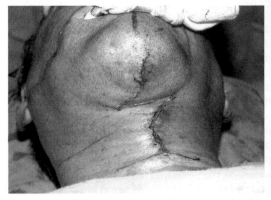

Fig. 8. Immediate postoperative view of anterior skin excision and z-plasty.

of the corset raise concerns regarding creation of a midline ridge. This is prevented by careful suturing, which prevents bunching of the platysma.

Lateral Platysma Window

Cruz and colleagues[32] described the platysma window. A reference point is made one fingerbreadth inferior to the angle of the mandible and one fingerbreadth anterior to the anterior border of the SCM muscle. Starting at this point, a 2 cm vertical incision is made in the platysma and a flap of platysma is raised, then spanning sutures are used to anchor the platysma flap to the mastoid fascia, posterior to the danger zone of the great auricular nerve.

Lateral Skin Displacement

This procedure was recently popularized by Mario Pelle-Ceravolo and colleagues.[1] Before this, the author performed a platysmaplasty and full-width platysma transection. One hundred fifty patients were observed for 1 year. They noted a high rate of recurrence of platysma banding (35.4%) and skin laxity (43.7%). The lateral skin displacement was designed to obviate these less-than-ideal results. Skin undermining is performed from lateral to medial and stops 6 to 7 cm from the midline. Then starting at a point 4 cm below the mandible, thus avoiding injury to the cervical branch of the facial nerve, a vertical incision following the platysma fibers is performed. This is followed by wide subplatysma undermining toward the midline. After creation of this subplatysma plane, the platysma is transected in a horizontal fashion creating upper and lower musculocutaneous flaps. These composite skin-muscle flaps are next sutured to the mastoid fascia using spanning sutures and avoiding injury to the great auricular nerve.

COMPLICATIONS

Long-term complications from the necklift operation include pixie ear, midline ridging, recurrent platysma bands, palpable or visible submandibular glands, facial nerve injury, and over- or underresection of fat. Short-term complications include hematoma formation.

An acutely expanding hematoma requires an immediate return to the operating room for evacuation and control of bleeding to prevent skin flap compromise and/or major airway problems.[33] A small hematoma discovered early in the postoperative period can be safely drained at the bedside.[34] A missed small hematoma can lead to formation of fibrous tissue that can lead to contour abnormalities. The incidence of hematoma after facelift surgery is reported at 1% to 11%,[33] and the most common risk factors include hypertension, aspirin and aspirin-like products, male gender, and anterior platysmaplasty.[35,36]

Hematomas after necklift surgery can be related to excision of the submandibular glands. Mendelson and Tutino[4] reported their experience with 112 patients. One patient needed emergent reoperation to evacuate a potentially fatal neck hematoma. The most frequent complications were temporary submandibular sialocele (4.5%) and temporary marginal mandibular neurapraxia (4.5%).[37] Resection of the submandibular glands for aesthetic reasons remains controversial.[38,39]

A pixie ear results from increased tension during closure of the periauricular incision, specifically at the level of the ear lobule. This complication can be prevented with cautious skin resection during facelift surgery at the level of the ear lobule, with the help of a Zins clamp or any other accurate measurement techniques. Repair of a pixie ear involves reopening of the skin incision and raising appropriate skin flaps, followed by closure under no tension with the ear lobule in the appropriate position.

During a corset platysmaplasty, the imbricating running sutures are placed lateral to the platysma edges to shorten the horizontal length of the muscle bilaterally and reduce the cervicomental angle. If the sutures are placed inappropriately, a ridge can be formed in the midline, which can be felt through the skin. This can be a source of frustration for both the patient and the surgeon and requires a trip to the operating room for correction.

Skin irregularities can be secondary to inadequate undermining. This is easily corrected in a second operation with adequate undermining performed. Less frequently, skin irregularities are related to undrained or inadequately drained seromas. This is usually hard to treat and best prevented by postoperative thoroughness.

Inadequate fat removal leads to contour irregularities. Undercorrection is usually treated in a second operation involving either liposuction or direct excision. However, overresection leading to skeletonization of the neck is hard to treat, highlighting the importance of conservative fat resection.

SUMMARY

Neck rejuvenation surgery should be meticulously tailored to the need of the patient to achieve a satisfactory result. It is now an integral part of facial rejuvenation with facelift, regardless of the platysma manipulation performed (**Figs. 9–13**).

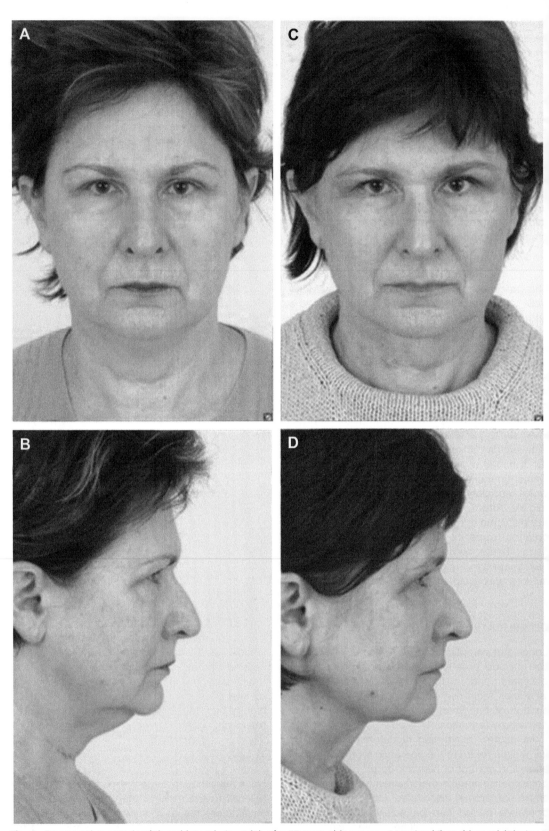

Fig. 9. Preoperative anterior (*A*) and lateral views (*B*) of a 57-year-old woman. Anterior (*C*) and lateral (*D*) views 1 year after anterior neck approach with anterior lipectomy and platysmaplasty and transconjunctival lower lid blepharoplasty.

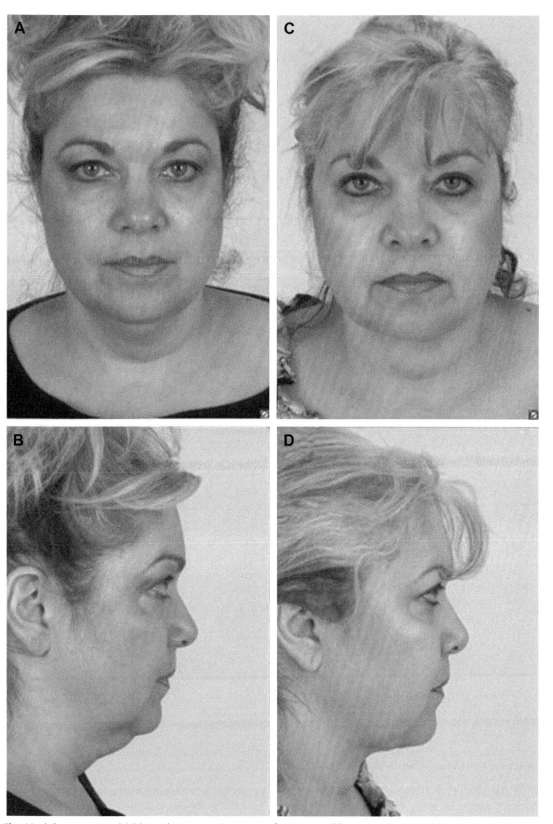

Fig. 10. (*A*) Anterior and (*B*) lateral preoperative views of a 50-year-old woman. Anterior (*C*) and lateral (*D*) views 1 year after anterior approach with liposuction, corset platysmaplasty, and resection of intermediate fat.

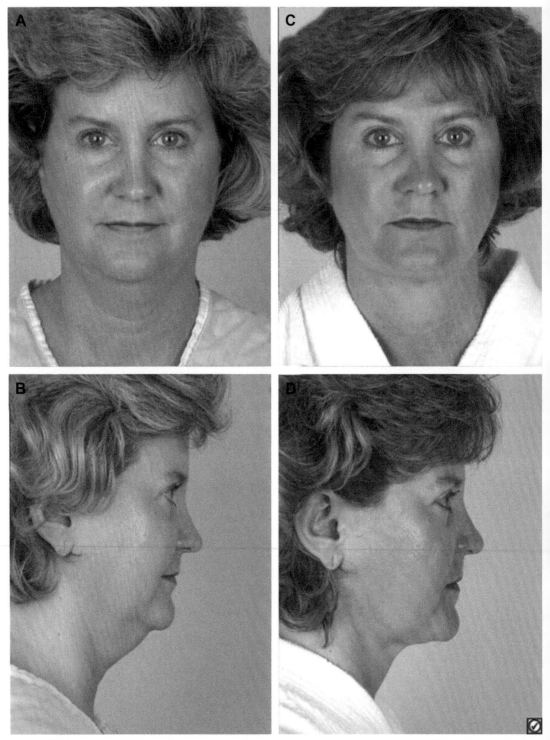

Fig. 11. (*A*) Anterior and (*B*) lateral preoperative views of a 43-year-old woman. Anterior (*C*) and lateral (*D*) views 1 year after anterior approach with liposuction alone.

When considering an isolated necklift, the most important factor to study is the amount of skin laxity in the neck. Young patients with grade II laxity are the best candidates for the anterior approach as adequate skin undermining will lead to appropriate skin contraction and redraping. Patients who have grade IV laxity are best treated with a standard face and necklift, as this will allow

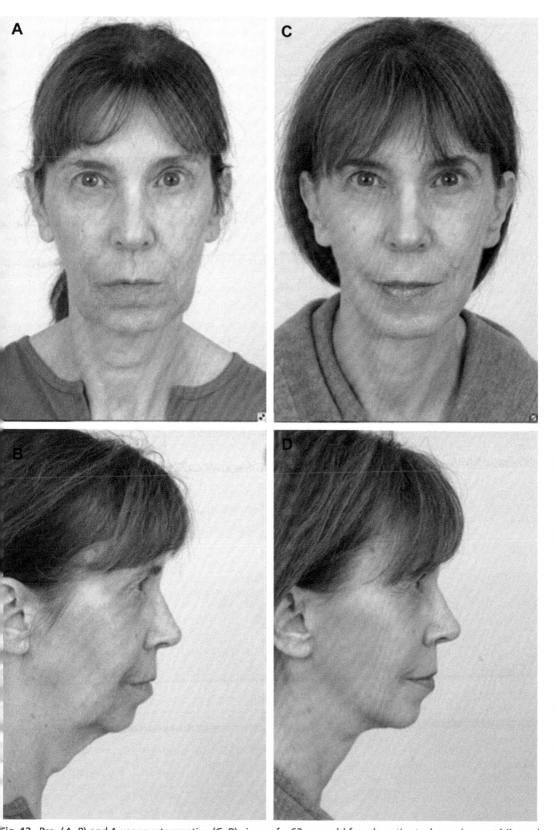

Fig. 12. Pre- (*A*, *B*) and 1-year postoperative (*C*, *D*) views of a 62-year-old female patient who underwent bilateral rhytidectomy with extended SMAS, perioral phenol-croton oil peel, and fat injections to the cheeks and nasolabial folds. A submental incision used to perform a pants-over-vest platysmaplasty.

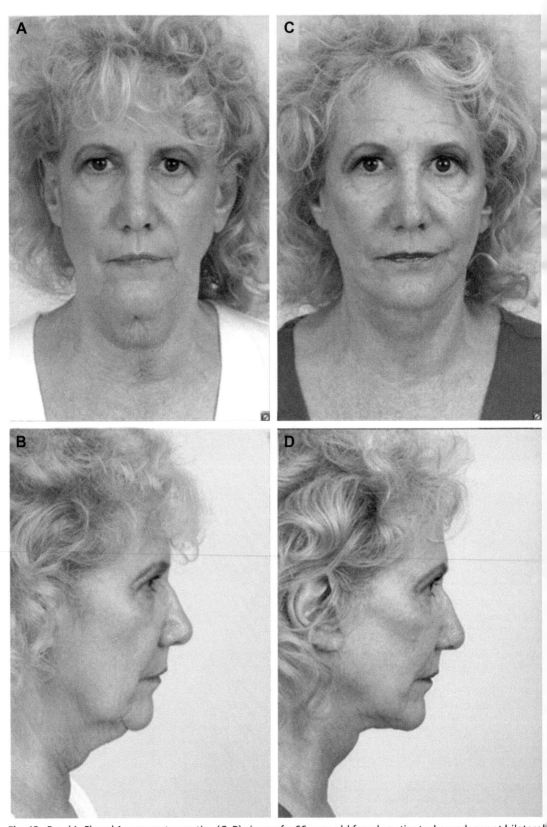

Fig. 13. Pre- (*A, B*) and 1-year postoperative (*C, D*) views of a 66-year-old female patient who underwent bilateral rhytidectomy with extended SMAS and fat injections to the cheeks and nasolabial folds. A submental incision used to perform a corset platysmaplasty and lipectomy.

for resection of the excess skin through the posterior neck incision.

An understanding of the three-dimensional anatomy of the neck, especially because it relates to the digastric muscles, fat compartments, and submandibular glands, is essential in tailoring the appropriate operation to the patient and in avoiding unhappy patients with mediocre aesthetic results.

SUPPLEMENTARY DATA

Supplementary data related to this article can be found online at https://doi.org/10.1016/j.cps.2019.06.004.

REFERENCES

1. Pelle-Ceravolo M, Angelini M, Silvi E. Treatment of anterior neck aging without a submental approach: lateral skin-platysma displacement, a New and proven technique for platysma bands and skin laxity. Plast Reconstr Surg 2017;139(2):308–21.
2. de Castro CC. The anatomy of the platysma muscle. Plast Reconstr Surg 1980;66(5):680–3.
3. O'Daniel TG. Understanding deep neck anatomy and its clinical relevance. Clin Plast Surg 2018; 45(4):447–54.
4. Mendelson BC, Tutino R. Submandibular gland reduction in aesthetic surgery of the neck: review of 112 consecutive cases. Plast Reconstr Surg 2015;136(3):463–71.
5. Feldman JJ. Surgical anatomy of the neck. Neck-lift. 1st edition. Stuttgart (Germany): Thieme; 2006. p. 106–13.
6. Furnas DW. The retaining ligaments of the cheek. Plast Reconstr Surg 1989;83(1):11–6.
7. Huettner F, Rueda S, Ozturk CN, et al. The relationship of the marginal mandibular nerve to the mandibular osseocutaneous ligament and lesser ligaments of the lower face. Aesthet Surg J 2015;35(2): 111–20.
8. Owsley JQ. Platysma-fascial rhytidectomy: a preliminary report. Plast Reconstr Surg 1977;60:843–50.
9. Tzafetta K, Terzis JK. Essays on the facial nerve: part I. Microanatomy. Plast Reconstr Surg 2010; 125(3):879–89.
10. Sinno S, Thorne CH. Cervical branch of facial nerve: an explanation for recurrent platysma bands following necklift and platysmaplasty. Aesthet Surg J 2019;39(1):1–7.
11. Trévidic P, Criollo-Lamilla G. Platysma bands: is a change needed in the surgical paradigm? Plast Reconstr Surg 2017;139(1):41–7.
12. Ozturk CN, Ozturk C, Huettner F, et al. A failsafe method to avoid injury to the great auricular nerve. Aesthet Surg J 2014;34(1):16–21.
13. Larson JD, Tierney WS, Ozturk CN, et al. Defining the fat compartments in the neck: a cadaver study. Aesthet Surg J 2014;34(4):499–506.
14. Zins JE, Menon N. Anterior approach to neck rejuvenation. Aesthet Surg J 2010;30(3):477–84.
15. Feldman J. My approach to neck lift. Denver (CO): Colorado Society of Plastic Surgeons; 1995.
16. Feldman J. Lesser lifts and ancillary procedures. Paper presented at the Annual Meeting of the American Society of Aesthetic Surgery. Orlando, FL, May, 1996.
17. Feldman J. The isolated neck lift. Paper presented at the Massachusetts General Hospital Aesthetic Symposium. Vail, CO, March, 1996.
18. Feldman J. Face or neck lift without a post auricular incision. Paper presented at the 33rd Annual Meeting of the American Society of Aesthetic Surgery. Orlando, FL, May, 2000.
19. Knize DM. Limited incision submental lipectomy and platysmaplasty. Plast Reconstr Surg 1998;101: 473–81.
20. Zins JE, Fardo D. The "anterior-only" approach to neck rejuvenation: an alternative to face lift surgery. Plast Reconstr Surg 2005;115:1761–8.
21. Ramirez OM. Cervicoplasty: nonexcisional anterior approach. Plast Reconstr Surg 1997;99:1576–85.
22. Courtiss EH. Suction lipectomy of the neck. Plast Reconstr Surg 1985;76:882–9.
23. Goddio AS. Skin retraction following suction lipectomy by treatment site: a study of 500 procedures in 458 selected subjects. Plast Reconstr Surg 1991;87:66–75.
24. Nahai F. Neck lift. In: Nahai F, editor. The art of aesthetic surgery: principles and techniques, Vol. II. St Louis (MO): Quality Medical Publishing, Inc.; 2005. p. 1239–83.
25. Guyuron B. Problem neck, hyoid bone, and submental myotomy. Plast Reconstr Surg 1992;90: 830–7 [discussion: 838–40].
26. Biggs TM. Excision of neck redundancy with single Z-plasty closure. Plast Reconstr Surg 1996;98: 1113–4.
27. Gradinger GP. Anterior cervicoplasty in the male patient. Plast Reconstr Surg 2000;106:1146–54 [discussion: 1155].
28. Kesselring UK. Direct approach to the difficult anterior neck region. Aesthetic Plast Surg 1992;16: 277–82.
29. Sullivan PK, Freeman MB, Schmidt S. Contouring the aging neck with submandibular gland suspension. Aesthet Surg J 2006;26:465–71.
30. Hamilton JM. Submental lipectomy with skin excision. Plast Reconstr Surg 1993;92:443.
31. Cronin TD, Biggs TM. The T-Z-plasty for the male "Turkey gobbler" neck. Plast Reconstr Surg 1971; 47:534.
32. Cruz RS, O'Reilly EB, Rohrich RJ. The platysma window: an anatomically safe, efficient, and easily

reproducible approach to neck contour in the face lift. Plast Reconstr Surg 2012;129(5):1169–72.

33. Schnur PL, Weinzweig J. A second look at the second-look technique in face lifts. Plast Reconstr Surg 1995;96(7):1724–6. Available at: http://www.ncbi.nlm.nih.gov/pubmed/7480299.

34. Grover R, Jones BM, Waterhouse N. The prevention of haematoma following rhytidectomy: a review of 1078 consecutive facelifts. Br J Plast Surg 2001; 54(6):481–6.

35. Baker DC, Aston SJ, Guy CL, et al. The male rhytidectomy. Plast Reconstr Surg 1977;60(4):514–22. Available at: http://www.ncbi.nlm.nih.gov/pubmed/909960.

36. Jones B, Grover R. Avoiding hematoma in cervicofacial rhytidectomy: a personal 8-year quest. Reviewing 910 patients. Plast Reconstr Surg 2004;113:381.

37. Singer DP, Sullivan PK. Submandibular gland I: an anatomic evaluation and surgical approach to submandibular gland resection for facial rejuvenation. Plast Reconstr Surg 2003;112(4):1150–4 [discussion: 1155–6].

38. Marten T, Elyassnia D. Short scar neck lift: neck lift using a submental incision only. Clin Plast Surg 2018;45(4):585–600 [Review].

39. de Pina DP, Quinta WC. Aesthetic resection of the submandibular salivary gland. Plast Reconstr Surg 1991;88(5):779–87 [discussion: 788].

Lateral Skin–Platysma Displacement
A New Approach to Neck Rejuvenation Through a Lateral Approach

Mario Pelle-Ceravolo, MD[a,b,*], Matteo Angelini, MD[b]

KEYWORDS

- Platysma bands • Neck rejuvenation • Excess cervical skin • Platysma transection
- Platysmectomy • Anterior neck flaccidity • Submandibular gland reduction

KEY POINTS

- Full neck undermining and complete platysma transection has been used for neck rejuvenation, with excellent immediate results but high rates of platysma bands and excess skin recurrence.
- Lateral skin–platysma displacement is based on a lateral approach to the neck, complete platysma transection and myocutaneous flaps and treats muscular bands and anterior skin laxity.
- Advantages of Lateral skin–platysma displacement include limited neck undermining, absence of submental scar, short operating time, fast patient recovery, satisfactory results, and easy approach for submandibular gland reduction.
- Lateral skin–platysma displacement has been shown to be an effective technique in terms of quality of results and low complication rates.
- Partial horizontal platysmectomy may be used in selected patients with very strong platysma bands, a more aggressive approach that may be more effective than Lateral skin–platysma displacement in certain cases.

OUR 25-YEAR EXPERIENCE IN TREATING NECK AGING

Skin laxity and platysma bands are the most common features of aging in the anterior neck area. The excess skin is usually confined to the lateral neck areas in younger people (<40 years old). In most older patients (>60 years old), overabundant skin accumulates, particularly in the anterior neck region. Skin laxity of the neck is commonly treated through skin–muscle undermining, traction applying specific vectors, and removal of overabundant tissue.

Platysma bands may be:

1. Hypertonic: the underlying muscle is thick and appears like a violin string, also when relaxed.
2. Hypotonic: the platysma is flaccid and thin.
3. Pseudobands: the bands consist only of a skin fold without muscle inside.

Hypertonic bands are the most difficult to eradicate and present a high recurrence rate despite aggressive treatments.

For more than 25 years (1983–2009), the senior author has used a technique based on complete neck undermining and full width platysma transection to treat platysma bands and anterior neck skin laxity.[1,2] In an article published in 2016, we evaluated recurrence rate of anterior skin laxity and platysma bands. At 1 year after surgery, 48% of patients showed recurrent anterior skin excess and 45% had recurrence of bands.[3] Owing to the disappointing results of this technique together

Disclosure Statement: The authors have nothing to disclose.
[a] University of Padua, Padua, Italy; [b] Private Practice, 35 Via Giovanni Severano, Rome 00161, Italy
* Corresponding author.
E-mail address: mario.pelleceravolo@live.it

Clin Plastic Surg 46 (2019) 587–602
https://doi.org/10.1016/j.cps.2019.06.006

with all the disadvantages of a complex operation, starting in 2010, we adopted a new technique,[4] namely, lateral skin–platysma displacement (LSD), using a different approach to the platysma without opening the anterior neck. This technique achieves very good results, decreases the operating time and complication rate, and provides a much faster postoperative recovery.

THE PRINCIPLES OF LATERAL SKIN–PLATYSMA DISPLACEMENT

This technique entails only a lateral approach without any submental incision and anterior neck undermining. The technique involved approaching the platysma on its midbody and not on its posterior border, undermining completely the muscle up to its medial border to render it mobile, transecting it horizontally, pulling the skin–muscle flap in a lateral direction, and then suturing it to the mastoid fascia using cable stitches. This maneuver would skew the anatomy of the platysma by relocating the muscle in a more lateral and horizontal position, thus strongly decreasing the risk of band recurrence.

Physics teaches us that the pulling effect of traction on elastic tissue decreases as the distance between the place where the traction is applied and the target area increases. Most classical techniques pull the skin or skin/muscle cervical flap from its lateral border to redrape the skin of the anterior neck.[5–15] This action has only a modest effect on remodeling the anterior neck skin, because the site where traction is applied is 12 to 14 cm away from the target area where the effect of the traction is desired (ie, the anterior neck). In contrast, exerting traction on the midbody of the platysma–skin flap, which is closer to the anterior neck, is more effective in treating the anterior skin laxity.

Moreover, pulling the platysma flap without undermining it, as we do during the full transection technique, means that the traction is exerted on a muscle that is adherent to the deep tissue, which means that, after it has been pulled laterally and sutured under tension, it will have a tendency to resume its previous position. In our approach, the wide undermining carried out on the muscle and the interruption of its continuity allow us to mobilize it freely and to displace it steadily in a more lateral position. This is done by tacking the muscle at a shorter distance from the midline, pulling it laterally together with the skin and suturing the myocutaneous flap to the mastoid fascia or the platysma-auricular ligament.

Owing to the effectiveness of the traction exerted on the midbody of the musculocutaneous

flap, the cervical skin is displaced laterally together with the muscle and this allows for the removal of a larger quantity of skin at the retroauricular area without exerting excessive tension on the cutaneous flap. Guerrerosantos and colleagues[16,17] and Gonzales[13,18] have published a technique based on a similar rationale but with different technical details.

When other factors are responsible for the unacceptable aesthetic appearance over the anterior neck (digastric muscles hypertrophy, presence of perihyoid fascia, etc), LSD is not the appropriate technique; other maneuvers necessitating an anterior approach would be indicated to treat each specific issue.[19–33]

SURGICAL TECHNIQUE

Preoperative markings were drawn with the patient in the upright position. The anterior vertical platysma bands were marked, and a 5-cm vertical line indicating the incision into the midbody of the platysma was drawn parallel and 6 to 7 cm lateral to the midline, keeping its upper end at 4 cm from the lower mandibular border. A horizontal line joining the previous 2 vertical lines was marked at 2 cm below the upper border of the thyroid cartilage to indicate the line of the platysma transection (**Fig. 1**).

After having prepared and infiltrated the area to be undermined with 250 mL of saline containing 20 mL of mepivacaine 2% and 2 mg of epinephrine, we carry out cutaneous undermining, which, in the neck area, extends to approximately 1.5 cm beneath the marked vertical incision on the platysma. Thus, approximately 5 to 6 cm of

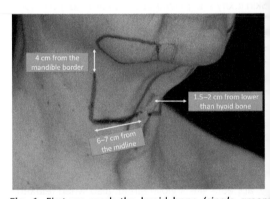

Fig. 1. First we mark the hyoid bone (*single green spot*), then the paramedian platysma band (*the vertical red line*), then the 5- to 6-cm-long vertical incision on the platysma (*the lateral vertical blue line*) at 6 to 7 cm from the midline, then the platysma transection line from the bottom of the vertical incision on the platysma to a point that is 1.5 to 2.0 cm lower than the hyoid bone.

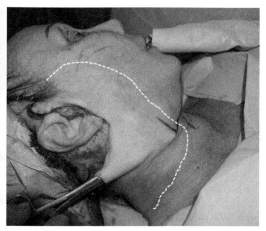

Fig. 2. The cervical skin flap is undermined up to 5 to 6 cm from the midline. The undermining overcomes about 1.5 cm of the vertical incision on the platysma.

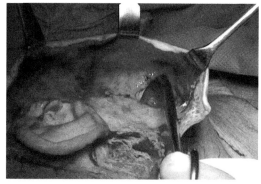

Fig. 4. The subplatysma undermining is carried out beyond the medial border of the muscle. Medially to the vertical line the whole platysma is still attached to the skin.

anterior neck skin on each side are not undermined and remain attached to the platysma (Fig. 2).

After obtaining good hemostasis, we make a 5- to 6-cm vertical eyelet using a Metzenbaum scissor on the platysma parallel to its fibers, following the preoperative marking that is 1 cm lateral to the limit of the cutaneous undermining. The highest point of this incision is never closer than 4 cm to the mandibular border to avoid any injury to the mandibular branch (Fig. 3). A horizontal tunnel under the muscle is carried out by spreading the scissors in the subplatysmal plane to reach a point beyond the medial border of the anterior platysma band (Fig. 4).

We undermine the platysma from lateral to medial bluntly, taking care not to injure the facial vein, which is frequently visible underneath the muscle at the level of the posterior border of the submandibular gland. This maneuver is essential to obtain an adequate mobilization of the platysma. Then we insert a slim retractor under the muscle to check that no muscular tissue is left behind and to avoid injury to any structure deep to the muscle. We divide the platysma in its full thickness horizontally to its medial border, ensuring that all medial platysma fibers were sectioned (Figs. 5 and 6). Once the platysma has been mobilized we carry out the traction of the myocutaneous flap.

DIFFERENT VECTORS OF TRACTION

The vector of traction may vary, resulting either in a posterior (LSD P; Fig. 7) or in a vertical vector (LSD V; Fig. 8). When we opt for LSD P, we pass a suture of a 3-0 PDS into the mastoid aponeurosis. The needle then takes a solid bite into the lower platysma flap and then is passed again into the mastoid aponeurosis (at approximately 5 cm behind and 10–12 cm below the tragus) in an area posterior to the course of the greater auricular nerve. The suture is not tied at this time. A

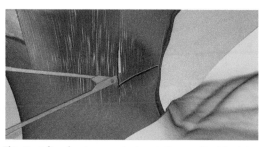

Fig. 3. After having carried out the vertical incision on the platysma at 4 cm lower than the mandibular border to avoid the risk of injuring the mandibular nerve, the scissors start the subplatysmal undermining.

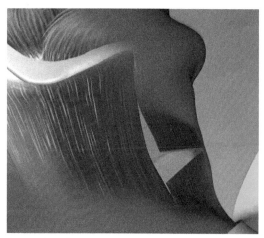

Fig. 5. The platysma is completely transected from its lateral incision to its medial border.

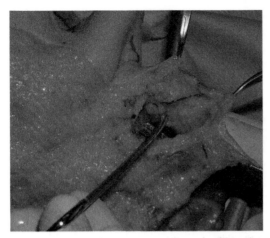

Fig. 6. Inspecting the transection line, checking that no muscular fibers has been left behind. Medially to the vertical incision line the platysma is still attached to the skin.

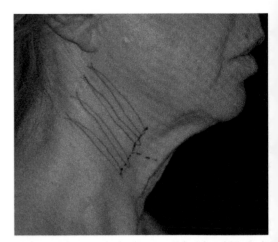

Fig. 9. Cable sutures (represented by the skin markings) are used (owing to the long distance between the myocutaneous flap and the mastoid aponeurosis) to avoid excessive tension and "cheese wiring."

second similar suture is placed to reinforce the first between the lower flap and a site 1.0 to 1.5 cm cranial than the first one on the mastoid fascia. One or 2 additional sutures are placed between the upper platysma flap and mastoid 1.0 to 1.5 cm cranially to the previous ones. At the end of suturing, we pull on the sutures to evaluate the adequateness of the traction.

Because the platysma does not reach the mastoid aponeurosis we use cable sutures to hold the muscle in position (**Fig. 9**). Once the 4 sutures are in place, they are tied, starting with the lower ones, securely but not tightly to avoid cheese wiring the muscle (**Fig. 10**).

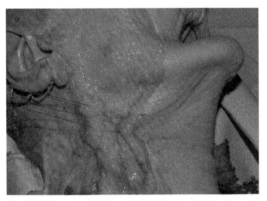

Fig. 7. The composite skin-platysma flap may be pulled through a horizontal vector and attached to the mastoid fascia (LSD P).

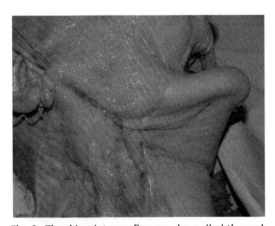

Fig. 8. The skin-platysma flap may be pulled through a vertical vector and attached to the platysma-auricular fascia (LSD V).

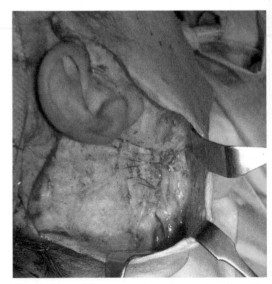

Fig. 10. The cable sutures have been placed on the patient.

When we opt for an LSD V, the upper flap is anchored on the platysma-auricular, about 2 cm caudad to the tragus and the lower flap is anchored to the mastoid fascia.

Each suture is passed back and forth (catching first the mastoid fascia or the platysma–auricular ligament, then the platysma, and again the mastoid fascia or the platysma–auricular ligament), leaving approximately 1 cm of space between the 2 threads to decrease the amount of fat bulging through the sutures. Sometimes fat protruding between the sutures is treated by cauterization.

The choice between the 2 vectors is based on the anatomy of the cervicomandibular area. LSD V has more power in defining the cervicomandibular angle but creates a certain fullness below the mandibular angle, whereas LSD P has less power on the cervicomental angle but achieves a better outlining of the mandible line and avoids any excess volume over the submandibular area. In patients in whom the submandibular gland is already visible and no reduction is planned, LSD P is usually the selected option. When in doubt, we try both vectors and then choose the one that shows the best result.

TECHNICAL VARIATIONS

The level of platysma transection may vary according to the patient's features and mainly to the presence of lower cervical skin flaccidity. In a patient without low cervical skin flaccidity the transection line starts at about 9 cm from the mandible and ending at 2 cm below the hyoid bone and only one myocutaneous flap is used for traction (LSD 1).

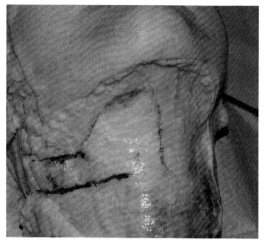

Fig. 12. In a specimen. On the right side, the LSD has been carried out whereas on the left side nothing has been done. Very little platysma is left on the right side of the anterior neck because the muscle has been displaced laterally. On the opposite, untreated side, the whole platysma is on the anterior neck.

This is the most frequently used technique at the present time. When lower neck cutaneous laxity is present the transection line is higher, starting at about 7 cm from the mandible and ending at 2 cm below the hyoid bone and 2 myocutaneous flaps are confectioned and (LSD 2). The strong traction on the mobilized platysma skews the alignment of the muscular fibers and moves the muscle away from the anterior neck, displacing it laterally (Fig. 11). Little platysma is left over the anterior neck, which explains why this technique entails a low risk of band recurrence (Fig. 12).

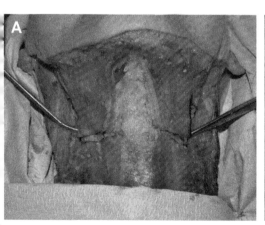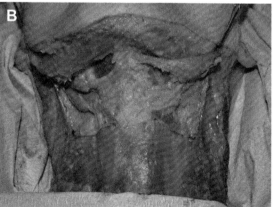

Fig. 11. (A, B) In a specimen. (A) The platysma has been incised vertically and transected horizontally. (B) If the platysma has been completely undermined from the deep cervicalis fascia, it can be easily pulled laterally and displaced from the anterior neck.

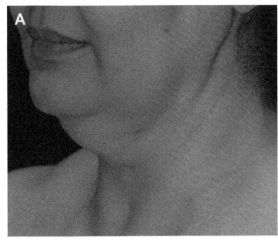
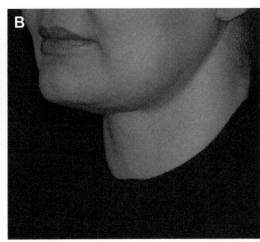

Fig. 13. (*A*, *B*) Preoperative appearance. A 57 year-old woman showing a fat neck with excess skin. No visible bands. (*B*) At 6 months after LSD, associated supraplatysmal and subplatysmal liposuction is performed. Improvement of the cervicomandibular angle with satisfactory skin remodeling is evident.

Because the platysma maintains its attachments to the skin of the anterior neck, traction on the platysma creates a powerful pull on the anterior neck skin, which is displaced laterally. Moving the excess skin closer to the mastoid area facilitates the removal of a larger amount of skin on the retroauricular area without tension.

The lateral portion of the platysma is mostly left undisturbed unless some lateral platysma bands require treatment. In this case, we remove a horizontal strip of the lateral platysma starting from its lateral border at 5 to 6 cm from the lower mandibular border to avoid injury to the mandibular nerve, which runs more cranially to this point.

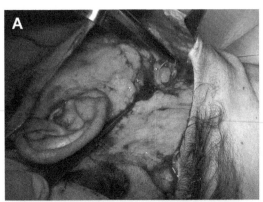
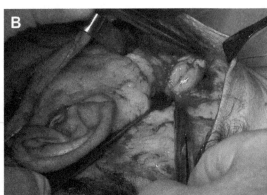
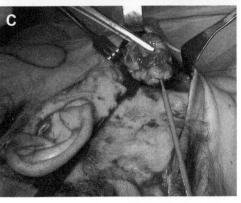

Fig. 14. (*A*) The forceps hold the capsule of the submandibular gland that has been opened through a lateral approach. (*B*) The gland has been widely freed so that it can be easily mobilized to allow effective hemostasis and reduction. (*C*) A large piece of the submandibular gland is removed.

In patients with excess fat over the anterior neck, liposuction is performed at the beginning of the procedure, that is, before the skin undermining phase. Superficial liposuction is carried out through a small incision in the submental fold. Subplatysmal liposuction is done after the tunnel under the muscle has been created through the same tunnel or through a minimal submental incision (**Fig. 13**).

SUBMANDIBULAR GLAND REDUCTION

Submandibular gland reduction is disliked by many surgeons who consider it too aggressive to be combined with a facelift. In our opinion, which is shared by many other authoritative colleagues,[4,5,11,29–31] this treatment is indicated in a considerable number of patients (about 30%–35% of our patients), and in many of them, it represents a conditio sine qua if satisfactory results are to be obtained. Even slightly visible glands preoperatively may become obvious after neck contouring maneuvers. The horizontal incision on the platysma carried out by the LSD exposes the submandibular gland and constitutes an easy approach for gland reduction (**Fig. 14**).

For many years we have carried out gland reduction through a submental approach.[6,7,9,18–20] Indeed, from 2010 onward, we began to use the retro-auricular transplatysmal approach routinely to reduce the gland (**Fig. 15**), because we found that it offers numerous advantages compared with a submental approach:

- Wider exposure
- Easier hemostasis
- Faster execution
- Absence of submental scar
- No risk of compressing hematoma.

When submandibular gland reduction is carried out through the lateral approach, the submandibular space is in continuity with the anterior neck owing to the horizontal platysma split. In the case of hemorrhage, the blood collection will not remain in a

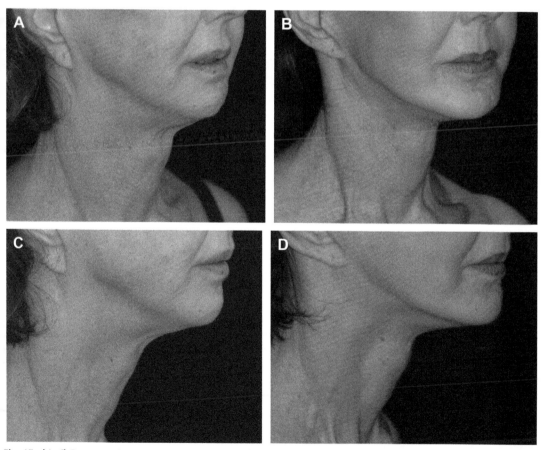

Fig. 15. (*A, C*) Preoperative appearance. A 63 year-old woman with moderate skin laxity and obvious submandibular gland protrusion. (*B, D*) Postoperative appearance 18 months after LSD P-1 with submandibular gland reduction and secondary mentoplasty. A good cervicomandibular angle was achieved. The gland treatment is mandatory in such a case to obtain an adequate neck contour.

closed space creating compression on the airways, because it may occur when the SMG is approached through a submental incision and the platysma is closed over the gland, but will spread into the anterior neck and can be treated like a neck hematoma avoiding life-threatening situations.[20]

NEW PROMISING IDEAS

Although LSD is a powerful procedure, in patients with considerable excess skin, we still have some disappointments owing to recurring anterior skin excess. Over the last 2 years, we have been using a different technique based on the use of a powerful cyanoacrylate glue that can create instant adhesion between the skin flaps and the deep tissues, allowing us to ameliorate the result of our traction maneuvers on the skin.

In some patients with overabundant anterior skin, a modified variation of LSD is carried out. The neck is widely undermined in the subcutaneous plane up to 2 to 3 cm from the midline. The platysma muscle, which, in this case, has no more adherence to the skin, is transected and sutured, as described regarding LSD.

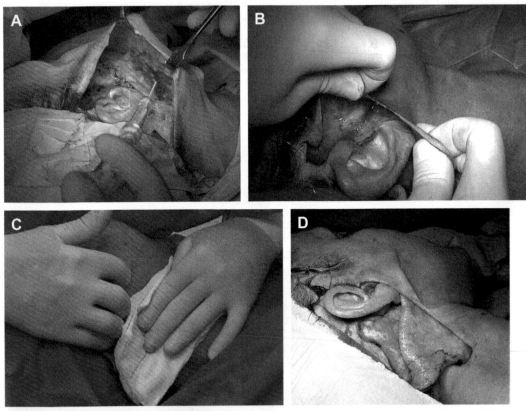

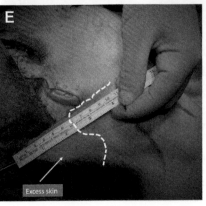

Fig. 16. (A) The glue is sprayed under the cutaneous flap. (B) The flap is strongly pulled following the selected vector. (C) Ninety seconds of compression is exerted on the flap. (D) The skin flap has completely adhered to the deep tissues. (E) A large amount of skin can be removed without any tension on the tip of the flap owing to the adherence created by the glue.

Eventually, this consists in a 2-planes facelift out with lateral platysma displacement. When we are ready for the flap traction, we apply a layer of glue on the surfaces of the flaps and of the deep tissues, through its specific sprayer device (**Fig. 16**A), we then strongly pull the flap following the selected vectors (**Fig. 16**B) and apply pressure for 90 seconds to let the glue polymerize (**Fig. 16**C). This creates immediate adhesion between the skin flap and the deep tissue (**Fig. 16**D). The progressive tension created by the glue on the medial area of the flap enhances the effectiveness of the traction on the lateral flap enabling the surgeon to remove a larger amount of skin (**Fig. 16**E) with no tension on the suture line. Cyanoacrylate glue is much more powerful than any fibrin glue; besides having analogous benefit in terms of sealing and hemostasis, the former has also a great capacity in fixating the flaps and holding the traction.

In some patients with strong hypertonic platysma, who are at higher risk for bands recurrence, we carry out a segmentary resection of the platysma as shown in **Fig. 17**, instead of using the LSD technique. This technique entails:

a. A wide subtotal subcutaneous and a limited subplatysma undermining (**Fig. 18**A, B),
b. The removal of a 4 to 5 cm wide strip of platysma from its lateral to its medial border (**Fig. 18**C–E),
c. Suturing the upper platysma flap to the mastoid area with a posterior and slightly oblique vector (**Fig. 19**A–H),
d. Using the glue to create a strong traction on the anterior skin flap.

This technique has been rendered effective by the use of the glue that fulfills the physical principles on which the LSD is based that is, the closer to the target area is the point of traction, the more effective is the traction.

DISCUSSION

All techniques based on complete neck undermining[1,2,5–7,9,19,21–33] entail certain risks, such as blood flow impairment, perioral muscular disturbances, visible irregularities, and certainly a long recovery, owing to the extensive undermined area in some cases (leather neck). Another drawback of full neck undermining is that a certain number of patients cannot be treated with this technique owing to other factors, such as smoking (**Fig. 20**), different therapies, and skin conditions that increase the risk of long flaps.

The length of the postoperative recovery period is one of the most important factors influencing the patient's decision in our practice. The patients' happiness is frequently related to the time necessary to return to a normal working or social life (**Fig. 21**). In our opinion, the full neck undermining technique is becoming anachronistic, because it constitutes an extended withdrawal from normal life, a condition that is either hardly acceptable or possible for many patients. Furthermore, after reviewing the results of our study on the outcome of neck-plasty technique based on full platysma transection, we were disappointed by our long-term results regarding the recurrence of platysma cords and anterior skin laxity, especially considering the aggressiveness of the technique used.

After a large experience with LSD, we are now routinely offering it to our patients presenting with moderate platysma bands and cervical skin laxity. The main advantages of LSD are[3,4]:

- Partial neck undermining means less operative time and potentially less risk.
- No submental scar.
- Good results in treating platysma bands and anterior skin laxity in a large number of our patients.
- It has been shown that LSD produces a notable decrease in the length of the postoperative recovery period of the LSD procedure when compared with other techniques with similar results.
- Our 9-year experience with this technique confirmed a very high patient satisfaction rate and an extremely low complication rate.

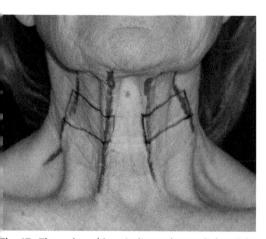

Fig. 17. The red markings indicate the medial and the lateral platysma borders. The blue markings outline the areas of the platysma to be removed.

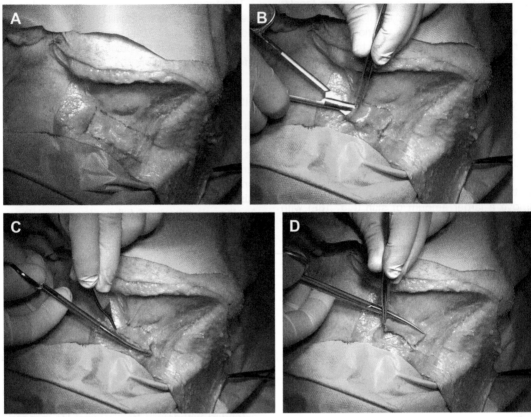

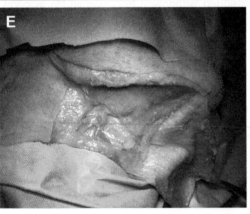

Fig. 18. In a specimen. (*A*) The skin and the subcutaneous fat have been removed and the platysma is exposed. The blue marking outlines the area that will be removed. (*B*) The scissors undermine the outlined area. (*C*) The scissors cut following the lower border of the marking. (*D*) The scissors cut following the upper border of the marking. (*E*) The muscular area has been removed exposing the sub-platysmal fat.

- An evaluation carried out on our patients, which showed that at 1 year the recurrence rate of platysma bands and, to a lesser extent, of anterior neck skin laxity is lower in patients treated with the LSD technique compared with the full neck undermining technique.
- It allows an easier reduction of the SMG through the retroauricular approach than through the submental approach.

There are some patients in whom LSD cannot achieve optimal results:

- Patients who present considerable amount of subcutaneous fat in the anterior neck. In these individuals, the aggressive liposuction over the anterior neck, necessary to obtain a good cervicomandibular angle, would destroy most of the attachments between the platysma and the skin, rendering the traction on the myocutaneous flap less effective.
- Patients with extensive and abundant subplatysmal fat. Despite suction carried out through the lateral subplatysmal incision can remove

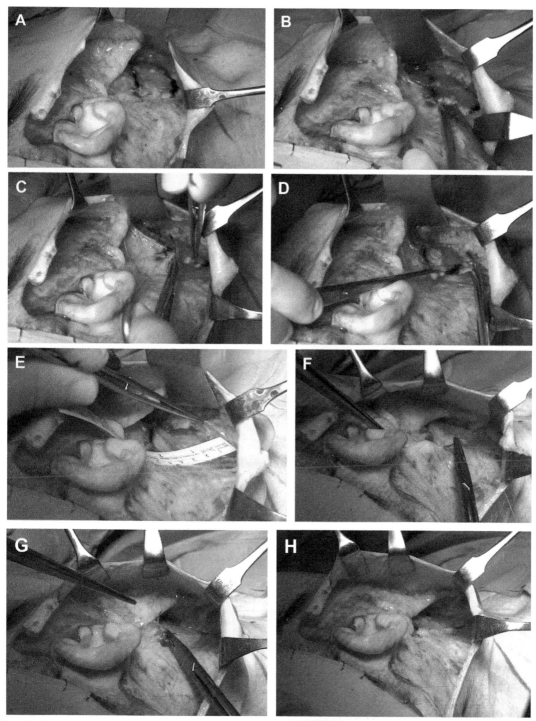

Fig. 19. The same maneuvers in a patient. (*A*) Undermining has been carried out in the juxtaplatysmal plane, leaving the subcutaneous tissue attached to the skin flap. The blue marking outlines the area that will be removed. (*B*) The scissors undermine the outlined muscular area beyond the medial platysma border. (*C*) The scissors cut following the upper border of the marking. (*D*) The scissors cut following the lower border of the marking. (*E*) The removal of the muscle interrupts the continuity of the platysma and a large (7–8 cm) gap creates between the 2 muscular stumps due to the muscle retraction. (*F*) A suture is passed through the mastoid aponeurosis. (*G*) The suture catches the upper platysma flap. (*H*) The suture is tied and the platysma flap is pulled and securely attached to the mastoid fascia.

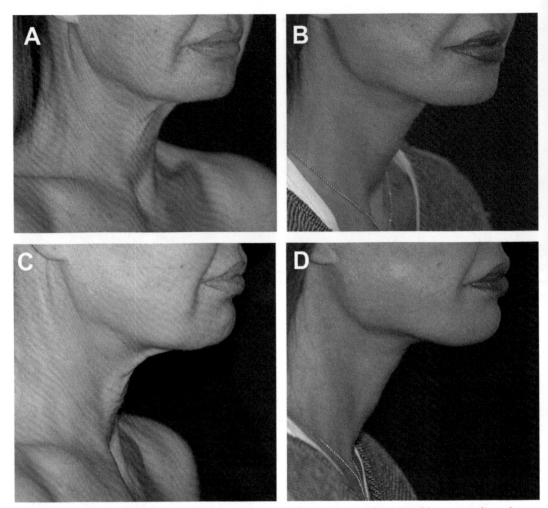

Fig. 20. (*A, C*) Preoperative. 55-year-old female heavy smoker patient with noticeable paramedian platysma bands at rest and anterior excess skin. (*B, D*) 1 year p-o- after LSD.

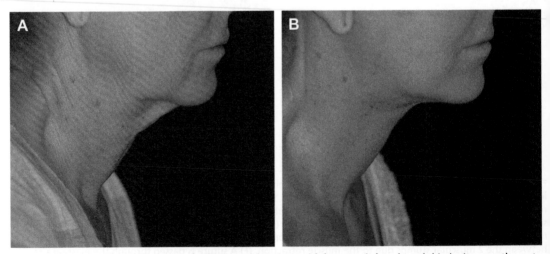

Fig. 21. (*A*) Preoperative appearance of a 58-year-old patient with hypotonic bands and skin laxity over the anterior neck. This patient refused SMG reduction (*B*) 1 year after LSD. Despite the visible presence of a bulging SMG, the cervical contour has substantially improved.

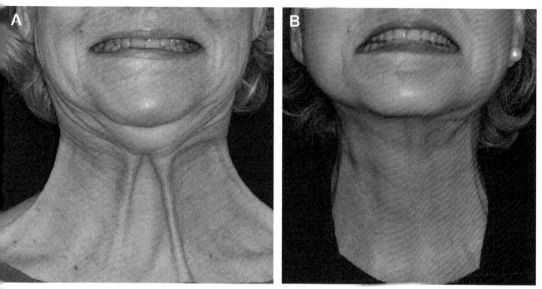

Fig. 22. (A) Preoperative appearance of a 65-year-old patient under forced platysma contraction. Hypertonic paramedian and lateral platysma bands are obvious. (B) Appearance at 1 year postoperatively after PHP (Partial Horizontal Platysmectomy). Under forced platysma contraction. Absence of platysma bands.

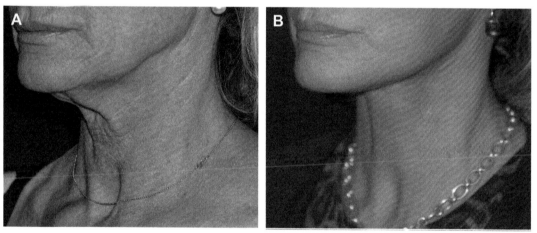

Fig. 23. (A) A 67-year-old woman with obvious platysma bands and lax skin on the anterior neck. (B) Appearance at 18 months after Partial Horizontal Platysmectomy. No bands are visible and a good cervical contoured has been restored.

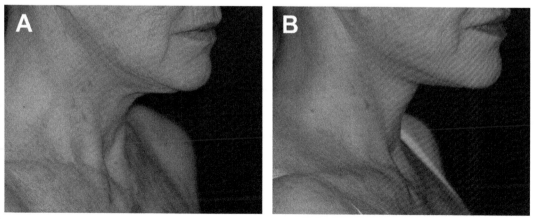

Fig. 24. (A) Preoperative. 65 y-o- female patient (S/P rhytidectomy 10 years before) with moderate amount of anterior excess skin and fat, platysma bands and ill-defined neck contour. (B) 18 months postoperative after atypical LSD with full neck undermining and glue application. The cervico-mandibular angle is nicely contoured, with absence of redundant skin.

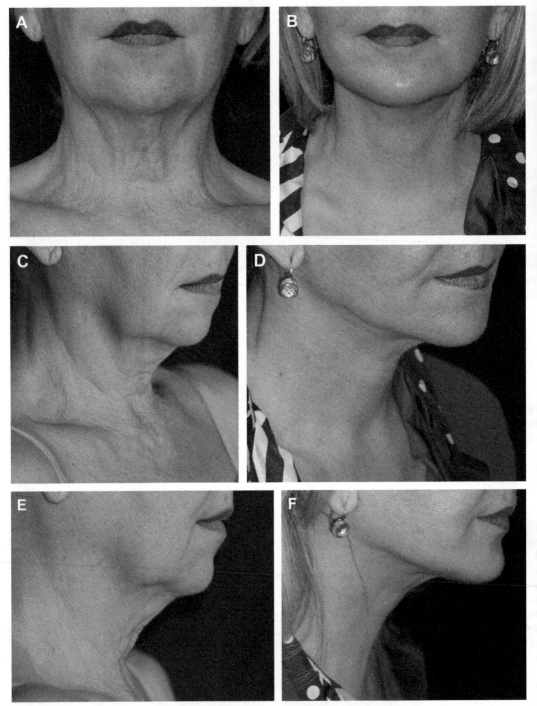

Fig. 25. (*A–F*) Preoperative appearance of a 65-year-old patient with anterior skin laxity, hypotonic platysmal bands, and supraplatysmal and subplatysmal fat excess. (*B, D, F*) Appearance at 1 year postoperatively after an LSD procedure and chin augmentation with implant. There is definite improvement of the bands, laxity, and general neck contour through the lateral approach.

much of this fat, and a more precise sculpturing can be obtained through a submental incision.

- When digastric hypertrophy is present a submental approach is necessary to shave or to remove the digastric muscles.

- In very difficult necks, that is, necks with anteriorized hyoid bones, frozen necks, or secondary situation with irregularities of the contour.

In these patients, an anterior approach is indicated to obtain satisfactory results. Furthermore, n some patients with very strong platysma bands (**Fig. 22**), we have used in the last 2 years a new technique named PHP (Partial Horizontal Platysmectomy), which entails the removal of a large strip of platysma in a horizontal direction together with the anchoring of the muscle flap to the mastoid aponeurosis. This technique, despite being more aggressive than LSD, because it necessitates a complete neck undermining carried out only through a lateral approach, has been shown to be very effective so far (**Figs. 23** and **24**). We are deepening our experience on this technique and will be publishing the results when an adequate follow-up will be available.

The adjunctive use of the cyanoacrylate glue constitutes is, in our opinion, a powerful tool in treating anterior skin laxity, one of the greatest challenges in neck rejuvenation.

SUMMARY

Currently, patient demands include not only the surgical outcome, but also the length of postoperative recovery period. The duration of the period in which patients must put aside their normal life constitutes a critical issue in making treatment decisions. This is one of the important reasons why many patients opt for simpler and easier solutions, which are often inappropriate for treating important deformities, especially in the neck.

Neck rejuvenation is a very challenging issue. Several authors have lately emphasized the importance of maneuvers directed to achieve good cervical contouring through aggressive lipectomy, reduction of the submandibular gland and of the digastric muscles in the majority of patients. This approach can produce precise neck sculpturing but, in our opinion, should not be applied indiscriminately to all patients, because it is an aggressive solution that entails a long postoperative recovery and a certain risk of complications.

LSD represents, in our opinion, a technique that can achieve satisfactory results with low complication and recurrence rates, and can be carried out successfully in 85% to 90% of the candidates for neck rejuvenation (**Fig. 25**).

Until 2011, we opened the neck in approximately 65% of our patients during a cervicofacial facelift and this number decrease to approximately 10% to 15% owing to the advantages provided by the LSD technique, which has now become our technique of choice in neck rejuvenation.

REFERENCES

1. Connel BF. Cervical lift. Surgical correction of fat contour problems combined with full platysma muscle flaps. Aesthet Plast Surg 1978;1(1):355–62.
2. Pelle - Ceravolo M, Botti G. Surgical treatment of the aging neck. Midface and neck aesthetic plastic surgery. 1st edition. Firenze (Italy): Acta Medica Edizioni; 2013. p. 838–926.
3. Pelle - Ceravolo M, Angelini M, Silvi E. Complete platysma transection in neck rejuvenation: a critical appraisal. Plast Reconstr Surg 2016;138: 781–91.
4. Pelle - Ceravolo M, Angelini M, Silvi E. Treatment of anterior Neck ageing without a submental approach: lateral skin-platysma displacement, a new and proven technique for platysma bands and skin laxity. Plast Reconstr Surg 2017;139(2):308–21.
5. Nahai F. Neck lift. In: Nahai F, editor. The art of aesthetic surgery: principles and techniques. 2nd edition. St Louis (MO): Quality Medical; 2011. p. 1675–715.
6. Feldman JJ. Neck lift. St Louis (MO): Quality Medical; 2006.
7. Feldman JJ. Corset platysmaplasty. Plast Reconstr Surg 1990;85(3):333–43.
8. Fogli A. The majority of necks can be corrected without a submental incision or anterior platysma procedures. Paper presented at: The Cutting Edge 2013 Aesthetic Surgery Symposium. New York, NY, December 6, 2013.
9. Marten TJ, Feldman JJ, Connel BF, et al. Treatment of the full obtuse neck. Aesthet Surg J 2005;25(4): 387–97.
10. Friel MT, Shaw RE, Trovato MJ, et al. The measure of face-lift patient satisfaction: the Owsley Facelift Satisfaction Survey with a long-term follow-up study. Plast Reconstr Surg 2010;126:245–57.
11. Millard DR Jr, Mullin WR, Ketch LL. Surgical correction of the fat neck. Ann Plast Surg 1983;10(5): 371–85.
12. Hamilton MM, Chan D. Adjunctive procedures to neck rejuvenation. Facial Plast Surg Clin North Am 2014;22(2):231–42.
13. Gonzales R. The LOPP-lateral overlapping plication of the platysma: an effective neck lift without submental incision. Clin Plast Surg 2014;41(1): 65–72.
14. Baker DC. Minimal incision rithydectomy (short scar face lift) with lateral SMAS-ectomy: evolution and application. Aesthet Surg J 2001;21:14.
15. Baker DC, Nahai F, Massiha H, et al. Short scar face lift. Aesthet Surg J 2005;25(6):607–17.
16. Guerrerosantos J, Espaillat L, Morales F. Muscular lift in cervical rhytidoplasty. Plast Reconstr Surg 1974;54:127.
17. Guerrerosantos J. Managing platysma bands and the aging neck. Aesthet Surg J 2008;28:211–6.

18. Gonzales R. Composite platysmaplasty and closed percutaneous platysma myotomy: a simple way to treat deformities of the neck caused by ageing. Aesthet Surg J 2009;29:344–54.

19. Marten TJ. High SMAS facelift: combined single flap lifting of the jawline, cheek and midface. Clin Plast Surg 2008;35(4):569–603.

20. Mendelson BC, Tutino R. Submandibular gland reduction in aesthetic surgery of the neck: review of 112 consecutive cases. Plast Reconstr Surg 2015;136:463–71.

21. Guyuron B, Sadek EY, Ahmadian R. A 26-year experience with vest-over-pants technique platysmarrhaphy. Plast Reconstr Surg 2010;126:1027–34.

22. Stuzin JM. Extended SMAS technique in facial rejuvenation. In: Nahai F, editor. The art of aesthetic surgery: principles and techniques. 2nd edition. St Louis (MO): Quality Medical; 2011. p. 1471–509.

23. Stuzin JM. MOC-PSSM CME article: face lifting. Plast Reconstr Surg 2008;121(Suppl):1–19.

24. Aston SJ. Platysma-SMAS cervicofacial rhytidoplasty. Clin Plast Surg 1983;10(3):507–20 [Review].

25. Hodgkinson DJ. Five-year experience with modified Fogli (Loré's fascia fixation) platysmaplasty. Aesthetic Plast Surg 2012;36:28–40.

26. Rosenfield LK. The pinch rhytidectomy: a safe, effective, "low SMAS" variation on the theme. Aesthet Surg J 2014;34:825–40.

27. Connell BF. Pushing the clock back 15 to 20 years with facial rejuvenation. Clin Plast Surg 2008;35:553–66.

28. Barton F. Facial rejuvenation. St Louis (MO): Quality Medical; 2008.

29. Stuzin JM, Baker TJ, Gordon HL, et al. Extended SMAS dissection as an approach to midface rejuvenation. Clin Plast Surg 1995;22:295–311.

30. Stuzin JM. Restoring facial shape in face lifting: the role of skeletal support in facial analysis and midface soft-tissue repositioning. Plast Reconstr Surg 2007;119:362–76 [discussion: 377].

31. Baker TJ, Stuzin JM. Personal technique of face lifting. Plast Reconstr Surg 1997;100:502–8.

32. Baker TJ, Gordon HL, Stuzin JM. Surgical rejuvenation of the face. 2nd edition. St Louis (MO): Mosby; 1996.

33. Feldman JJ. Neck lift my way: an update. Plast Reconstr Surg 2014;134:1173–83.

Facial Anatomy for Filler Injection

The Superficial Musculoaponeurotic System (SMAS) Is Not Just for Facelifting

Christopher C. Surek, DO[a,b,c,d],*

KEYWORDS

- Facial fat compartments • Superificial musculoaponeurotic system (SMAS) • Facial artery
- Angular artery • Superficial temporal artery • Pre-zygomatic space
- Deep lateral chin fat compartment • Osseocutaneous ligaments

KEY POINTS

- The prezygomatic space is a desirable target for deep augmentation of the lateral cheek.
- The deep medial cheek fat compartment and deep pyriform space can be used to soften the nasolabial fold and peripyriform shadow.
- Key landmarks and surface topography can be used to identify and potentially avoid the main trunk and associated branches of the facial artery as it traverses through the face.
- Injection into the deep medial chin fat compartment is a desirable target for chin augmentation with volume.
- The deep lateral chin fat compartment can be volumized to soften a prominent prejowl sulcus shadow.

INTRODUCTION

The Fear of Injections, is the Fear of Anatomy
—Adapted from Ian Taylor's 1982 quote
"The Fear of Surgery, is the Fear of Anatomy"

In the spirit of this facelift edition of *Clinics in Plastic Surgery*, this article journeys through facial anatomy for the injector with a specific emphasis on utilization of the superficial musculoaponeurotic system (SMAS) as a unique tool for the facial injector. The SMAS is a structure that is familiar to the facelift surgeon and induces a mental image that can be applied to injectable procedures throughout the face.

The role of volume augmentation with filler and/or fat has become increasingly important in facial aesthetic rejuvenation. Whether the surgeons themselves are performing the injections or extenders of the surgeon are performing the procedure, the tenants remain the same; strive for optimal results and avoid complications. The American Society of Aesthetic Plastic Surgeons statistics reported 722,394 injections in 2017 and this number continues to increase. There has been a 40% increase in injectables over the past 5 years.[1,2] Looking back even further, there has been a 312% increase in minimally invasive procedures from 2000 to 2017.[3]

In contrast with facelift surgery where the surgeon can directly visualize the structures being treated, facial injection is often a blind stick, leaving the injector to estimate depth and location based on surface topography and experience.

Disclosure: The author is a consultant for Allergan, Galderma and Cypris Medical.
[a] Kansas City University, Kansas City, KS, USA; [b] University of Kansas Medical Center, Kansas City, KS, USA; [c] Department of Plastic Surgery, Cleveland Clinic, Cleveland, OH, USA; [d] Private Practice, Surek Plastic Surgery, Overland Park, KS USA
* 7901 W. 135th Street, Overland Park, KS 66223, USA.
E-mail address: csurek@gmail.com

Therefore, this inability for injectors to directly visualize anatomic targets is why anatomic accuracy is critical to avoid suboptimal outcomes.

The objective of this article is to illustrate the layered anatomy in each facial aesthetic subunit and demonstrate high yield pearls that can be used by the facelift surgeon when performing volumizing procedures. The overarching concept is depth. The face is a 3-dimensional structure with lymphatic, neurovascular, and ligament networks, all of which can come into play when performing injections.

To navigate facial depth in the face the author suggests thinking of the facial layers in each aesthetic subunit as the supra-SMAS and the sub-SMAS, thereby facilitating a comprehensive categorization of the fat compartments, potential spaces, ligaments, lymphatics, and neurovascular networks in 2 distinct planes. Particular emphasis will be given to the facial vasculature because vascular compromise is one of the most dreaded complications of facial injection. In the worst of instances, this complication can lead to skin necrosis and blindness.[4-8]

THE TANGO BETWEEN THE SUPERFICIAL MUSCULOAPONEUROTIC SYSTEM (SMAS) AND THE FACIAL VASCULATURE

Described by Mitz and Peyronie[9] in 1976, the SMAS has been a cornerstone of facial rejuvenation for decades. In the modern day this structure can now play an integral role in non-surgical volumization of the face. Joel Pessa[10] teaches that the SMAS is a vestigial remnant of the pan-facial muscles of lower primates and explains that the SMAS acts as a highway to traffic important structures (mainly vessels and motor nerves) around the face. In many regions of the face, the facial vasculature demonstrates an intimate relationship with the SMAS, particularly in the jawline, perioral, nasolabial fold, infrabrow, and temple regions.[11-16] Therefore, using these principles as a baseline the injector can navigate superficial and deep to the SMAS while potentially avoiding interactions with facial vasculature in the process.

A suggested analogy of this concept is the middle layer of a 2-tiered cake. The platter that the cake sits on is analogous to the facial skeleton. The middle layer of icing (ie, the SMAS) is the center point, with a layer of cake below it (ie, sub-SMAS, preperiosteal, deep fat, and potential spaces) and a layer of cake above it (ie, supra-SMAS, subcutaneous) and then topped with icing (ie, the skin; **Fig. 1**). Consider this analogy as we take a journey through key facial aesthetic subunits.

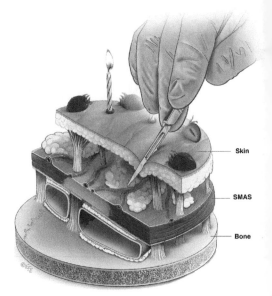

Fig. 1. Concept diagram for the layered anatomic arrangement in the face. Demonstrating the SMAS as a central layer with categorized structures deep and superficial containing fat compartments and potential spaces for target volumization. (*Courtesy of* Levent Efe, CMI, Melbourne, Australia.)

MIDFACE AND TEAR TROUGH
Sub-SMAS (Subsuperficial Musculoaponeurotic System)

The sub-SMAS midface has been a well described target for cheek volumization.[3,11,12] For the purposes of anatomic classification, the deep midface can be divided into upper and lower components partitioned by the zygomaticocutaneous ligaments. This imaginary division line has been termed the malar equator (**Fig. 2**).[11,13]

The lower sub-SMAS midface contains the deep medial cheek fat compartment and deep pyriform space. An additional potential space, the premaxillary space has been identified but has yet to be shown as a preferred target for cheek augmentation.[3,11-15]

The deep medial cheek fat compartment lies on the anterior maxilla and is divided into medial and lateral segments by the levator anguli oris muscle. Medial to this fat compartment lies the deep pyriform space. This space lies adjacent to the pyriform aperture. The angular artery has been described to traverse lateral and superficial to this space; however, vascular anatomy in this region can be variable (**Fig. 3**).[17]

The deep pyriform space and deep medial cheek fat compartments lie underneath the lip elevators, which are contained within the SMAS; therefore, clinical volumization of these targets helps to soften the nasolabial fold prominence

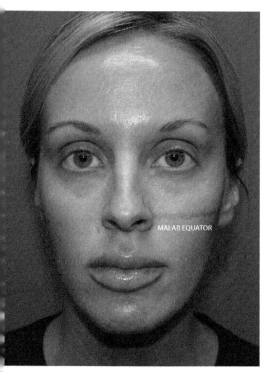

Fig. 2. Photograph of a model demonstrating the malar equator, a topographic landmark for the approximate location of the zygomaticocutaneous ligaments.

and peripyriform shadowing. Access to this space has been demonstrated through a variety of insertion points within a 1.5-cm area of the alar base (**Fig. 4**).[11,13–15]

The upper sub-SMAS midface contains the suborbiculairs oculi fat, preperiosteal fat, and the prezygomatic space. The preperiosteal fat pad is described as a thin fat pad residing on the surface of the zygoma. The suborbicularis oculi fat (SOOF), by definition, lies on the undersurface of the orbicularis muscle. A potential gliding space exists between these two fat compartments, termed the prezygomatic space. This space has been well-described as a target for cheek volume restoration. The prezygomatic space is bordered superiorly by the orbital retaining ligament and inferiorly by the zygomaticocutaneous ligaments. These ligaments coalesce medially at the tear trough ligament. Laterally, the space is bordered by the lateral orbital thickening. The far lateral extent of the zygomaticocutaneous ligaments is the main zygomatic ligament (**Fig. 5**). When using cannula, injectors will often feel a palpable and even audible pop as they traverse through the SMAS into the prezygomatic space. This is a confirmatory sign of safe passage into the sub-SMAS upper midface.[11]

Of note, the deep chain of facial lymphatics courses from the lower eyelid into the floor of the prezygomatic space before descending in the

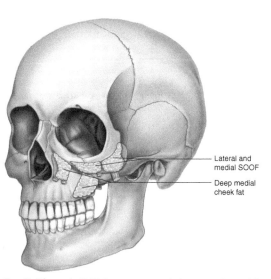

Fig. 3. The sub-SMAS structures of the anterior midface. The deep medial cheek fat compartment is divided into medial and lateral components by the levator anguli oris muscle. Adjacent to the pyriform aperture is the deep pyriform space. SOOF, suborbicularis oculi fat.

Lateral and medial SOOF

Deep medial cheek fat

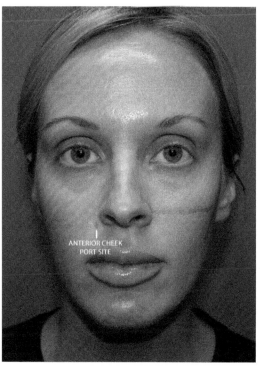

Fig. 4. Port insertion for access to the deep anterior midface volumization targets.

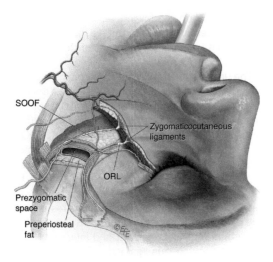

Fig. 5. The sub-SMAS structures of the lateral midface. The preperiosteal fat pad resides on the body of the zygoma. The suborbicularis oculi fat (SOOF) lies on the undersurface of the orbicularis oculi muscle. Between these 2 fat compartments is the prezygomatic space. Note the ligamentous boundaries of the space, the orbital retaining ligament and zygomaticocutaneous ligaments. The lymphatic and vascular networks are also displayed. (*Courtesy of* Levent Efe, CMI, Melbourne, Australia.)

lower midface.[18] The angular vasculature predominantly lies medial to the prezygomatic space and the tear trough ligament. A topographic marking 1.7 cm from midline and 1.3 cm inferior to the medial canthus has been described as an approximate location of the angular artery.[11,19] However, aberrant angular vessels have been described in up to 30% of cadaver samples. The course of this aberrant system is more lateral within the nasojugal groove. Topographically, this difference corresponds with a point 3.5 cm lateral from the midline, level with the supratip break and converging with the midpupillary line[19] (**Fig. 6**). The angular vein has been mapped 4.2 mm ($\pm$0.7) inferior to the infraorbital foramen coursing superomedially deep to the orbital leaf of the orbicularis oculi muscle.[3]

Supra-SMAS (Suprasuperficial Musculoaponeurotic System)

The supra-SMAS midface consists of superficial fat that is divided by vascularized septae creating distinct compartments. These compartments include the nasolabial, medial superficial, middle superficial, and lateral temporal cheek compartments[12] (**Fig. 7**). During cannula injection in the subcutaneous plane of the submalar hollow, resistance is often readily felt as the cannula traverses from one compartment to the next.[11] In the aging face, the depression that extends inferiorly from

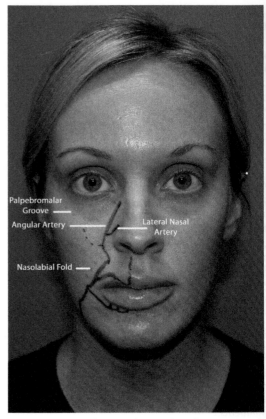

Fig. 6. Topographic markings for the commonly described facial and angular artery trajectories in the midface.

the tear tough into the cheek is titled the nasojugal groove and has been noted to result from volume shifts in the nasolabial and medial cheek fat compartments.[12]

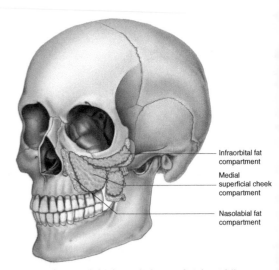

Fig. 7. The nasolabial, medial superficial, middle superficial, and lateral temporal cheek fat compartments.

The most superior superficial fat compartment in the midface is the infraorbital or malar fat compartment.[12] This compartment is straddled by the cutaneous insertions of the orbital retaining ligament (superiorly) and the zygomaticocutaneous ligaments (inferiorly). The superficial lateral chain of lymphatics course through this compartment. Iatrogenic malar mounds from filler injection have been documented in the literature and disruption of this lymphatic chain may be a contributing factor to this phenomenon.[11,13]

Based on the described anatomy, superficial volumization of the midface fat compartments in the submalar hollow can be a desirable technique to expand the cheek and overall facial proportions, however superficial volumization of the upper midface between the cutaneous insertions of the orbital retaining ligament and zygomaticocutaneous ligament should be approached with caution because there is the potential for lymphatic disruption in this plane.[11,13]

PERIORAL AND NASOLABIAL FOLD
Sub-SMAS (Subsuperficial Musculoaponeurotic System)

The facial artery ascends over the mandibular border coursing just lateral and often deep to the depressor anguli oris (ie, the sub-SMAS). It continues into the perioral region intimate with the modiolus complex giving off the inferior and superior labial vessels. In the majority of instances, these vessels remain deep to the orbicularis muscle (ie, the sub-SMAS) as they traverse medially. This path may traverse the supra-SMAS plane in the philtrum or central lower lip in a smaller percentage of people.[20–24] Owing to this principle, many lip injections are performed in the supra-SMAS plane in the upper lip, philtrum and lower lip. The idea behind this approach is to maximize the return on the investment of volume and topographic alteration while attempting to avoid vascular complications.[25] Authors have described potential spaces in the subvermillion (ie, supra-SMAS) of the upper and lower lip that can be readily accessed with cannulas for lip augmentation.[11,26]

The inferior labial artery comes off the facial artery within an area 2.4 cm from the oral commissure and 2.4 cm superior to the lower border of the mandible traversing submucosal to the midline. The path of the artery is variable; the main trunk can travel as low as the labiomental crease or has high as the vermillion cutaneous junction.[20,21] The superior labial artery is not always a bilateral structure. Studies have shown that up to 43% of subjects had 1 superior labial

artery. The branching of the superior labial artery off of the facial artery is generally in a 1.5 cm^2 area from the oral commissure at a depth of approximately 3.5 mm. The artery will commonly traverse cephalic the white roll for the lateral two-thirds of the lip and then dive caudal to the white roll at the proximal third of the lip at a depth of 3 mm as it terminates in the median tubercle of the upper lip. From there, the artery gives off an ipsilateral philtral branch[22] (**Fig. 8**). The philtral branch is suborbicularis 75% of the time; however, data has shown that the artery can travel superficial to the muscle in 25% of studied specimens.[27]

The facial artery then ascends from the perioral region medial to the nasolabial fold and most commonly crosses the fold at an average depth of 5 mm at the junction of the middle and proximal third of the fold.[11,28] It is at this point where there often seems to be an intimate relationship of the angular artery and the SMAS (see **Fig. 8**). This relationship seems logical since the artery's path courses through the insertions of SMAS into the nasolabial fold.[29–32] The SMAS and the angular artery are often interlaced until the artery approaches the region of the alar crease where it most commonly traverses subcutaneous as it gives of the lateral nasal artery. It then courses in the alar facial groove to anastomose with the dorsal nasal artery.

This vessel pattern is the reason several published resources suggest deep preperiosteal

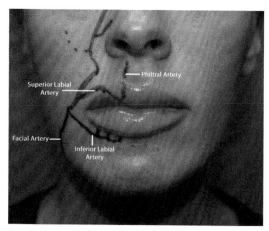

Fig. 8. Topographic markings for inferior labial, superior labial, and facial artery. Note the superior labial courses cephalic to the white roll for the lateral two-thirds of the ipsilateral upper lip and then traverses caudal to the white roll into the medial tubercle of the lip in the proximal third at an average depth of 3 mm. Then, a philtral artery branches vertical and superior toward the columella. The facial artery travels medial to the nasolabial fold and then crosses beneath the fold at the proximal third at an average depth of 5 mm.

injections on the bone in the anterior cheek and intradermal or immediate subdermal injection in the nasolabial fold. Additionally, studies recommend exercising caution in superficial injections in the peripyriform shadow because the depth of the angular artery at this level seems to be variable and less predictable.[16,33] To summarize, in the anterior cheek staying supra-SMAS in the nasolabial fold and sub-SMAS in the pyriform region are likely to be safe planes to help decrease the incidence of vascular injury (**Fig. 9**).

The main deep fat compartment of interest in the upper lip is the retro-orbicularis oris fat. As the name suggests, this compartment resides deep to the orbicularis oris muscle. It has been postulated that this fat compartment loses turgor with age and authors have postulated volumization of this compartment for perioral rejuvenation.[11]

Supra-SMAS (Suprasuperficial Musculoaponeurotic System)

Superficial fat compartments of the lip have been described; however, given the strong fibrous network between the perioral skin and the underlying musculature, this fat can be dispersed and vary in thickness, density, and demarcation. Three distinct boundaries define the subcutaneous boundaries of the perioral region: the nasolabial sulcus, the labiomental sulcus, and the submental sulcus. Volume augmentation in this region should be approached carefully and product selection is paramount, given the dynamic interplay of muscle and skin with animation.[3]

JAWLINE AND CHIN
Sub-SMAS (Subsuperficial Musculoaponeurotic System)

The sub-SMAS jawline contains the deep medial and lateral chin compartments as well as the mandibular osteocutaneous retaining ligament (MOCL) and platysma mandibular ligament (PML). Similar to the midface, these ligaments can act as boundaries of injection when performing volume correction of the prejowl sulcus.[11]

The PML is located approximately 5 cm distal to the gonial angle and acts as a fulcrum of stability for the platysma as it contracts over the jawline. The PML is analogous to the zygomaticocutaneous ligaments in that it possesses a hammock-like effect to help prevent injected volume to descend below the jawline into the neck. Additionally, the PML is analogous to the orbital retaining ligament owing to its stabilizing function on the platysma muscle (**Fig. 10**).[34]

The MOCL resides 5.6 cm distal to the gonial angle and 1 cm above the mandibular border. The

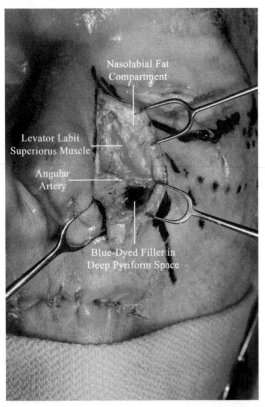

Fig. 9. Cadaveric dissection demonstrating blue dyed hyaluronic acid filler within the deep pyriform space and adjacent anatomic structures. Note the location and path of the latex injected angular artery vessels.

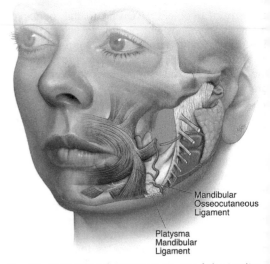

Fig. 10. Pertinent sub-SMAS anatomy of the jawline. The mandibular osseocutaneous ligament, PML, deep medial, and deep lateral chin fat compartments. (*Courtesy of* Levent Efe, CMI, Melbourne, Australia.)

igament has been described as spanning 3.6 mm n width and interdigitates with the depressor anguli oris muscle. Therefore, the MOCL contributes to the lower marionette fold and is a transition point between the anterior jowl and marionettes.[34]

The deep chin fat contains medial and lateral compartments. The medial compartment lies on the mentum deep to the mentalis muscle and functions as a suitable target for deep chin augmentation. The deep lateral chin fat compartment lies deep to the depressor anguli oris muscle, facilitating muscle glide and has been described as a key injection target for volume correction of the prejowl sulcus (see **Fig. 10**).[11,12]

Several approaches to the prejowl have been described. The author's preferred approach is through a paramedian port via cannula injecting cephalic to the PML and caudal to the MOCL to volumize the deep lateral chin fat compartment. For injectors who prefer a more direct approach with a sharp needle, be mindful of the facial artery, which ascends over the jawline through the antigonial notch, delivering vessels within or along the undersurface of the depressor anguli oris muscle and then continuing cephalic to give off the inferior labial artery[11] (see **Fig. 10**; **Fig. 11**).

Supra-SMAS (Suprasuperficial Musculoaponeurotic System)

The supra-SMAS jawline contains the superior and inferior jowl compartments which are separated from the submandibular compartment by the cutaneous insertion of the PML. With aging, repeated gliding of the platysma over the mandible results in counter-clockwise shift of the compartments around the ligaments with gradual inferior descent. This leads to the commonly described stigmata of lower facial aging.[3,35,36]

TEMPLE
Sub-SMAS (Subsuperficial Musculoaponeurotic System)

The temple remains a controversial topic in the current realm of facial injections. To date, the question remains as to what is the best plane to inject. Certain authors target deep on the bone, others target superficial fat and, in some instances, intermediate targets are discussed.[11,37] A chronic issue with temple anatomy is that there are several different names for the same structure. Studies have attempted to simplify this.[38,39]

The etiology of the temple hollow has been well-studied and research shows that the anterior–inferior trough is the deepest part of the temporal fossa. In youth, this trough is camouflaged by bulky soft tissue; however, as the face ages, thinning of this soft tissue exposes the temple hollow, creating an aesthetic deformity.[40]

The deepest layer of fat in the temple is the temporal extension of the buccal fat pad (aka the deep temporal fat pad), which lies deep to the deep temporal fascia. Wedged between the 2 layers of deep temporal fascia is the intermediate temporal fat pad. Interestingly, the bulk of this quadrangular fat pad is focused in the anterior–inferior trough and studies show a volume loss with age in this compartment is a key component of aging the temple hollow. The intermediate temporal fat pad receives its

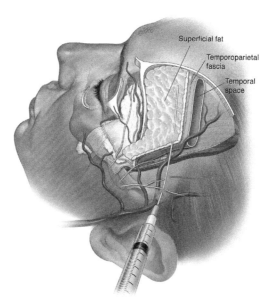

Fig. 12. Pertinent anatomy of the temple. Note the fat compartments of the temple and associated fascial layers along with the demonstration of the superficial temporal artery coursing within the temporoparietal fascia (ie, SMAS). (*Courtesy of* Levent Efe, CMI, Melbourne, Australia.)

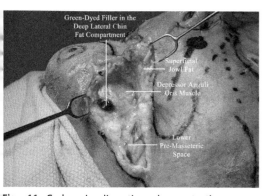

Fig. 11. Cadaveric dissection demonstrating green dyed hyaluronic acid filler deep lateral chin fat compartment. Note the relationship of the superficial jowl fat, depressor anguli oris and the facial artery branches relative to this sub-SMAS injection target.

vascular supply from the maxillary artery system (**Fig. 12**).

A potential space lies between the deep temporal fascia and the superficial temporal fascia titled the upper temporal space. This space is bordered superiorly by the superior temporal septum (STS) and inferiorly by the inferior temporal septum. A commonly described method of deep temporal augmentation is the use of an intersection point 1 cm superior along the STS and then 1 cm posterior to the STS with an injection directly on bone. Others have suggested adjusting this marking to 1.5 cm superior along the STS and 1.5 posterior to the STS[37] (**Fig. 13**).

Supra-SMAS (Suprasuperficial Musculoaponeurotic System)

The superficial temporal fascia is the SMAS equivalent in the temporal region. The superficial temporal artery travels within this fascia and often communicates with the orbital vascular system up to 70% of the time. This relationship between the superficial temporal artery and orbital vasculature is very important for each injector to understand as this has implications in vascular occlusions that can lead to blindness. The superficial temporal (subcutaneous) fat pad lies superficial to the superficial temporal fascia and is a common target for temporal volumization in the subcutaneous plane (see **Fig. 13**).

ORBIT

Periorbital injection is a hot topic in the current literature. As the specialty of plastic surgery transitions from a volume reduction era to the volume retention era in upper blepharoplasty the desire and necessity of infrabrow volumization is increasing.[41] However, detailed depictions of the periorbital vascularity are sparse. Actually, one can travel back to 1986 and credit Barry Zide and Glenn Jelks[42] with providing one of the first descriptions of tributaries stemming from the supraorbital and supratrochlear vessels. These tributaries can possess direct connections between the central retinal artery, the forehead and temple vasculature.

Anecdotally, many skilled surgeons demonstrate beautiful results from infrabrow injection. However, the question remains: What is the key to these surgeons avoiding vascular problems? A common port site is the lateral tail of the brow. The vessel that is in closest proximity to this port site is the supraorbital vasculature. In cadaveric dissection on a limited sample there appears to be an intimate relationship of the supraorbital tributary and the orbicularis muscle (**Figs. 14** and **15**). The SMAS envelopes the orbicularis on its anterior and posterior surface.[11] As is seen in other parts of the face, the vessels tend to run in and around this posterior lamella of SMAS. Therefore, the common description of hugging the orbital rim on the bone during infrabrow injection places the injection in a sub-SMAS plane and conceivably in a plane that may decrease the incidence of vascular injury. This is an important pearl considering the possible adverse sequelae of vascular compromise in this region (ie, blindness). However, more anatomic and clinical data is needed regarding the efficacy and safety of infrabrow volumization.

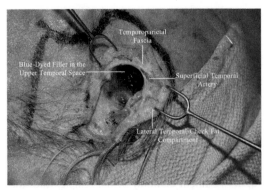

Fig. 13. Cadaveric dissection demonstrating blue dyed hyaluronic acid filler within the upper temporal space and adjacent anatomic structures. Note the location of the superficial temporal artery traveling within the temporoparietal fascia (ie, SMAS).

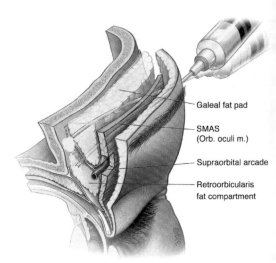

Fig. 14. The relationship of the SMAS, supraorbital arcade, retro-orbicularis fat compartment and galeal fat pad. (*Courtesy of* Levent Efe, CMI, Melbourne, Australia.)

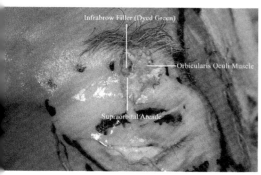

Fig. 15. Cadaveric dissection demonstrating green dyed hyaluronic acid filler within the retro orbicularis oculi fat compartment and adjacent anatomic structures. Note the location of the latex injected supraorbital vessel arcade running with the SMAS on the undersurface of the orbicularis oculi muscle.

SUMMARY

Facial volumization with filler and/or fat can serve as a finishing touch to compliment surgical repositioning of aging soft tissue. The depth of injection and anatomic awareness are paramount to help avoid vascular, lymphatic and other undesirable sequalae. Each aesthetic subunit can be approached in a systematic fashion to target sub-SMAS or supra-SMAS structures including fat compartments and potential spaces. This method can help the injector to obtain safe, accurate and aesthetically pleasing facial volume correction.

ACKNOWLEDGMENTS

The author would like to thank the Department of Anatomy at Cleveland Clinic, specifically Dr. Richard L Drake PhD and Dr. Jennifer McBride PhD. The author would like to acknowledge Levent Efe CMI for his hard work on the beautiful medical illustrations.

REFERENCES

1. Richards B, Schleicher W, D'Souza G, et al. The role of injectables in aesthetic surgery: financial implications. Aesthet Surg J 2017;37(9):1039–43.
2. 2017 procedure statistics. American Society for Aesthetic Plastic Surgery.
3. Cotofana S, Lachman N. Anatomy of the facial fat compartments and their relevance in aesthetic surgery. J Dtsch Dermatol Ges 2019;17(4): 399–413. Published by John Wiley & Sons LTD; 1610-0379.
4. Lazzeri D, Agostini T, Figus M, et al. Blindness following cosmetic injections of the face. Plast Reconstr Surg 2012;129:995–1012.
5. DeLorenzi C. Complications of injectable fillers, part 2: vascular complications. Aesthet Surg J 2014; 34(4):584–600.
6. Lee D, Yang H, Kim J, et al. Sudden unilateral visual loss and brain infarction after autologous fat injection into nasolabial groove. Br J Ophthalmol 1996; 80(11):1026–7.
7. Ozturk C, Li Y, Tung R, et al. Complications following injection of soft-tissue fillers. Aesthet Surg J 2013; 33:862–77.
8. Park T, Seo S, Kim J, et al. Clinical Experience with hyaluronic acid complications. J Plast Reconstr Aesthet Surg 2011;64:892–6.
9. Mitz V, Peyronie M. The superficial musculo aponeurotic system (SMAS) in the parotid and cheek area. Plast Reconstr Surg 1976;58(1):80–8.
10. Cosmetic corner interview with Joel Pessa MD, 2017. Available at: https://academic.oup.com/asj.
11. Lamb J, Surek C. Facial volumization: an anatomic approach. 1st edition. New York: Thieme Medical Publishers; 2017.
12. Pessa J, Rohrich R. Facial topography: clinical anatomy of the face. St. Louis (MO): Quality Medical Publishing; 2012.
13. Surek C, Beut J, Stephens R, et al. Pertinent anatomy and analysis for midface volumizing procedures. Plast Reconstr Surg 2015;135(5):818e–29e.
14. Surek C, Beut J, Stephens R, et al. Volumizing viaducts of the midface. Aesthet Surg J 2015;35(2): 121–35.
15. Surek C, Vargo J, Lamb J. Deep pyriform space: anatomical clarifications and clinical implications. Plast Reconstr Surg 2016;138(1):59–64.
16. Scheuer J, Sieber D, Pezeshk R. Facial danger zones: techniques to maximize safety during soft tissue filler injections. Plast Reconstr Surg 2017; 139(5):1103–8.
17. Gierloff M, Stohring C, Buder T, et al. Aging changes of the midfacial fat compartments: a computed tomographic study. Plast Reconstr Surg 2012; 129(1):263–73.
18. Shoukath S, Taylor I, Mendelson B, et al. The lymphatic anatomy of the lower eyelid and conjunctiva and correlation with post-operative chemosis and edema. Plast Reconstr Surg 2017;139(3):628–37.
19. Yang H, Lee J, Hu K, et al. New anatomical insights on the course and branching patterns of the facial artery: clinical implications of injectable treatments to the nasolabial fold and nasojugal fold. Plast Reconstr Surg 2014;133(5):1077–82.
20. Tansatit T, Apinuntrum P, Thavorn P. A typical pattern of the labial arteries with implication for lip augmentation with injectable fillers. Aesthetic Plast Surg 2014;38:1083–9.
21. Edizer M, Magden O, Tayfur V, et al. Arterial anatomy of the lower lip. Plast Reconstr Surg 2003;111(7): 2176–81.

22. Lee S, Gil Y, Choi Y, et al. Topographic anatomy of the superior labial artery for dermal filler injection. Plast Reconstr Surg 2015;135(2):445–50.

23. Crouzet C, Fournier H, Papon X, et al. Anatomy of the arterial vascularization of the lips. Surg Radiol Anat 1998;20(23):273–8.

24. Pinar Y, Bilge O, Govsa F. Anatomic study of the blood supply to the peri-oral region. Clin Anat 2005;18:330–9.

25. Loukas M, Hullett J, Louis R, et al. A detailed observation of variations of the facial artery, with emphasis on superior labial artery. Surg Radiol Anat 2006;28:316–24.

26. Pensler J, Ward J, Perry S. The superficial musculoaponeurotic system in the upper lip: an anatomic study in cadavers. Plast Reconstr Surg 1985;75(4):488–92.

27. Furukawa M, Mathes D, Anzai Y. Evaluation of the facial artery on computed tomographic angiography using a 64-slice multidetector computed tomography: implications for facial reconstruction in plastic surgery. Plast Reconstr Surg 2013;131(3):526–35.

28. Nakajima H, Imanishi N, Aiso S. Facial artery in the upper lip and nose: anatomy and clinical application. Plast Reconstr Surg 2002;109(3):855–61.

29. Beer G, Manestar M, Mihic-Probst D. The causes of the nasolabial crease: a histomorphological study. Clin Anat 2013;26:196–203.

30. Rubin L, Mishriki Y, Lee G. Anatomy of the nasolabial fold: the keystone of the smiling mechanism. Plast Reconstr Surg 1989;83:1–10.

31. Pessa J, Brown F. Independent effect of various facial mimetic muscles on the nasolabial fold. Aesthetic Plast Surg 1992;16:167–71.

32. Barton F, Gyimesi I. Anatomy of the nasolabial fold. Plast Reconstr Surg 1997;100(5):1276–80.

33. Fagien S, Fitzgerald R, Matarasso A. Soft tissue fillers and neuromodulators: international and multidisciplinary perspectives. Plast Reconstr Surg 2015;136(33):9S–10S.

34. Huettner F, Rueda S, Oztruk C, et al. "The relationship of the marginal mandibular nerve to the mandibular osseocutaneous ligament and lesser ligaments of the lower face". Aesthet Surg J 2015 35(2):111–20.

35. Lambros V. Observations on periorbital and midface aging. Plast Reconstr Surg 2007;120(5):1367–76.

36. Lambros V, Amos G. Three-dimensional facial averaging: a tool for understanding facial aging. Plast Reconstr Surg 2016;138(6):980–982e.

37. Lamb J, Martin A, Walker R, et al. Three dimensional CT validation of supraperiosteal temple volumization with hyaluronic acid filler techniques. Plast Reconstr Surg Glob Open 2018;(9 suppl):166.

38. O'Brien J, Ashton M, Rozen W, et al. New perspectives on the surgical anatomy and nomenclature of the temporal region: literature review and dissection study. Plast Reconstr Surg 2013;131(3):510–9. Discussion by Knize D. on 523-25.

39. Moss C, Mendelson B, Taylor G. Surgical Anatomy of the ligamentous attachments in the temple and peri-orbital regions. Plast Reconstr Surg 2000;105:1475–90 [discussion: 1491–98].

40. Vaca EE, Purnell CA, Gosain AK, et al. Postoperative temporal hollowing: is there a surgical approach that prevents this complication? A systematic review and anatomic illustration. J Plast Reconstr Aesthet Surg 2017;70(3):401–15.

41. Surek C. The SMAS is not Just for Facelifting Presentation at the Annual Meeting of the American Society of Aesthetic Plastic Surgeons. New Orleans, May 18, 2019.

42. Zide B, Jelks G. Surgical anatomy of the orbit. 1st edition. New York: Raven Press; 1985.

Nonsurgical Adjuncts Following Facelift to Achieve Optimal Aesthetic Outcomes: "Icing on the Cake"

Ziyad S. Hammoudeh, MD*, W. Grant Stevens, MD

KEYWORDS

• Facelift • Nonsurgical • Cosmetic medicine • Lasers • Intense pulsed light • Botulinum toxin
• Facial aging

KEY POINTS

- A facelift is effective at tightening laxity in the underlying support structures of the face/neck and removing redundant facial skin, but it is ineffective at treating other aging changes of the skin.
- Aesthetic outcomes following facelift surgery can often be optimized by the addition of nonsurgical adjuncts to achieve a more complete facial rejuvenation.
- Facial volume enhancement, skin resurfacing, intense pulsed light for pigmentary lesions, neuro-modulators, and skin care are all important components of maximizing the results of a facelift.
- Skin resurfacing can be successfully performed via dermabrasion, chemical peels, or lasers with each possessing advantages and disadvantages. The authors' treatment strategy for skin resurfacing with lasers following facelift is outlined.

INTRODUCTION

Facial aging can manifest as multiple different physical findings. These findings include loss of skin elasticity, laxity of support structures, volume deflation, rhytids (wrinkles), and sun damage with pigmentation and uneven texture. For a complete facial rejuvenation, each of these distinct manifestations must be treated in specific ways to achieve a more youthful appearance. Therefore, it is important to understand the pathophysiology of each of these manifestations as well as the surgical and nonsurgical options available to combat these signs of aging. That is where the interface of cosmetic medicine and surgery come together.[1]

A facelift combats both skin redundancy and laxity of the underlying support structures of the face, namely the superficial musculoaponeurotic system (SMAS) and platysma. Laxity of the underlying support structures leads to descent of the soft tissues in the lower third of the face and neck. Various techniques of tightening the SMAS have been described to lift the soft tissue, including SMAS excisions, plications, and flaps of different designs.[2] Multiple options also exist for addressing the platysma either beneath the skin flaps laterally or through a submental incision. However, a facelift has minimal effect on improving the quality of the skin other than removing redundancy.

The terms rhytidectomy and facelift are often used interchangeably. However, the nomenclature rhytidectomy (wrinkle removal) is actually a misnomer; although a facelift is effective at correcting laxity of the support structures and removing excess skin, it is not effective at removing fine rhytids from the remaining skin. A facelift also will not

Disclosure Statement: The authors have no disclosure of any relationship with a commercial company that has a direct financial interest in the subject matter or materials discussed in this article or with a company making a competing product.
Private Practice, Marina Plastic Surgery, 4644 Lincoln Boulevard, Suite 552, Marina Del Rey, CA 90292, USA
* Corresponding author.
E-mail address: ziyad.hammoudeh@gmail.com

Clin Plastic Surg 46 (2019) 613–623
https://doi.org/10.1016/j.cps.2019.06.002
0094-1298/19/© 2019 Elsevier Inc. All rights reserved.

improve the collagen content or elasticity of the skin, and it will not correct pigmentary changes. Therefore, other treatment modalities are needed to address these common coinciding signs of facial aging. Such treatments include volume enhancement of the underlying soft tissues, resurfacing of the skin to treat fine rhytids and uneven texture, phototherapy to treat pigmentary lesions, neuromodulators to block the muscles that lead to deep rhytids, and skin care to hydrate and nourish the skin. These adjuvant nonsurgical treatments following a facelift are the "icing on the cake" that helps achieve an optimal aesthetic outcome.

FACIAL VOLUME ENHANCEMENT

With age, the face loses volume in the form of fat atrophy and bone loss. Consequently, facial volume enhancement is needed in a large number of facelift patients to restore a youthful appearance. Autologous fat grafting has become very popular among plastic surgeons as the preferred method of facial volume rejuvenation during facelifts.[3] Advances in autologous fat grafting has led to the concept of the lift-and-fill facelift.[4,5] The concept of replacing a patients' lost facial fat with their own autologous fat from unwanted areas of their body has become very popular. Stem cells within the transferred fat also have the potential advantage of rejuvenating the overlying skin, thereby combating another factor contributing to the aged appearance. The disadvantages of fat grafting include some unpredictability of outcome because not all of the transferred fat will be retained, and there is the possibility of lumpiness or fat necrosis postoperatively.

Soft tissue volume enhancement can also be achieved with synthetic fillers postoperatively, particularly to areas in which palpability is more concerning, such as the lips, or for small refinements in volume of the cheeks, nasolabial folds, and temples as maintenance treatments after a facelift with fat transfer. Hyaluronic acid (HA) fillers are typically preferable for augmenting the lips because of their predictability and their smooth consistency with lower risk of palpability.[6,7] The disadvantage of HA fillers to the lips is the lack of permanence and required maintenance treatments over time. Surgical modalities for augmenting the lips other than fat grafting have also been used, including palmaris longus grafts,[8,9] SMAS grafts,[10] and alloplastic implants.[11,12] For patients who have a long upper lip in addition to a thin vermillion, a lip lift can also be considered to shorten the distance from the nasal base to the vermillion to address this concern in addition to volume enhancement.[13]

For patients who are very thin with minimal body adiposity for harvesting and limited fat recipient beds in the face to receive substantial volume, other options are available. In such cases, poly-L-lactic acid (PLLA) filler can be used postoperatively. PLLA is a semipermanent filler that stimulates collagen production and has been successful in treating patients with severe facial fat wasting.[14] Therefore, PLLA fillers may be preferable to HA fillers in some cases because of the long-lasting effect. For replacement of lost bone, such as the malar or chin region, calcium hydroxyapatite filler can be used to augment the skeletal structure postoperatively. Although less commonly used these days because of the advent of fillers and advancements in fat grafting, alloplastic facial implants are a reasonable option for either bony or soft tissue augmentation of the malar, chin, or temporal region in patients who are severely volume depleted.[15]

SKIN RESURFACING

Skin resurfacing involves removal of the superficial skin surface to expose healthy underlying layers as a treatment of rhytids, uneven texture, fine scars (eg, acne scars), large pores, and some sun damage. Rhytids involve varying depths of the skin layers depending on their severity. *Superficial* rhytids involve the epidermis; *medium* rhytids involve the *papillary* dermis, and *deep* rhytids involve the *reticular* dermis. Therefore, skin resurfacing depth of penetration is aimed at targeting the desired layer of involvement. The 3 main modalities of skin resurfacing include dermabrasion, chemical peels, and laser resurfacing. Each of these modalities has their own advantages and disadvantages.

There is a dual insult to the facial skin when a facelift is combined with simultaneous skin resurfacing. During a facelift, undermining of the subcutaneous flaps of facial skin eliminates the underlying perforators that run from deep to superficial in the z-axis toward the skin surface. The skin maintains perfusion via small arterioles and venules in the subdermal plexus running in the x–y-axis parallel to the surface with potential for impaired perfusion at the distal tips of the skin flaps. When there is a concomitant injury to the dermis from the superficial surface in addition to dissection on the deep surface subcutaneously, there is a potential for increased risk of skin necrosis. For this reason, the safety of resurfacing the undermined skin at the same time as a facelift is controversial and should be approached with caution. Resurfacing of the skin that is not undermined during a facelift, such as the perioral skin, considered very safe for resurfacing because the underlying perforators on the deep surface of the skin are preserved, so there is only a surface insult without a subcutaneous insult. Perioral wrinkles are very common with aging and are also common among smokers, so they should be evaluated for potential treatment with nonsurgical adjuncts following a facelift.

Dermabrasion

Dermabrasion involves the use of a hand-held rotating instrument to mechanically abrade the outer layers of aged skin to promote reepithelialization.[16] It removes the epidermis and penetrates into the papillary or reticular dermis. Perioral dermabrasion has long been an intraoperative adjunct in face-lifting. The advantages of using dermabrasion for skin resurfacing include the relatively inexpensive cost of the instrument with minimal maintenance costs over time. The disadvantage is a relative lack of precision of depth control and even distribution over the treatment area that is surgeon dependent. Control is particularly limited around curved surfaces of the face, such as the labiomental aspect of the perioral region.

Microdermabrasion is a less aggressive treatment that exfoliates the outermost layer of the epidermis without penetration into the dermis.[17] It uses a fine jet of aluminum oxide crystals to abrade the epidermis while a microvacuum removes the crystals and dead skin cells. Microdermabrasion is an in-office procedure that can be used as on-going skin maintenance following a facelift. However, it is infrequently used as an adjunct to face-lifting because of its less drastic effect compared with dermabrasion, chemical peels, and lasers, which are more aggressive resurfacing options that normally require recovery time but can be combined with face-lifting without producing additional recovery time beyond that needed for the facelift.

Chemical Peels

Chemical peels are categorized based on depth of penetration as either superficial, medium, or deep.[18] *Superficial* peels include alpha-hydroxy acids (lactic acid, glycolic acid, tartaric acid, or malic acid) or Jessner solution (salicylic acid + ethanol + lactic acid + resorcinol). *Medium*-depth peels include varying concentrations of trichloroacetic acid (TCA). Phenol croton oil peels offer the operating surgeon a great deal of flexibility. Although once considered a deep peeling technique only, Hetter has shown that this technique can be used as a superficial, intermediate, or deep peel, depending on the nature of the frost generated.[19,20] The

depth of penetration depends not just on the peel solution contents but also on the solution concentration, skin type, pretreatment preparation, application technique, and repetition frequency.[21] For instance, TCA concentrations of 35% to 50% function as a *medium*-depth peel, whereas concentrations of greater than 50% function as a *deep* peel. Chemically treated skin will turn *pink* initially and then develop a *white* frost on the surface because of coagulation of proteins, which signifies that penetration has reached beyond the epidermis into the papillary dermis. A *gray* hue indicates a deeper than desired level of penetration. The advantage of a chemical peel is the minimal expense of the chemical agent without other additional costs. The disadvantage is a relative lack of precise depth control and even distribution of the chemical agent over the treatment area that requires an experienced provider to determine when penetration depth is satisfactory. Therefore, chemical peels require the greatest clinical assessment to avoid complications.

In the 1960s, Baker[22] was among the first to combine chemical peels with face-lifting; he performed a phenol peel on the forehead only at the time of face-lifting and then applied the phenol peel to the remainder of the face approximately 3 weeks after the facelift because of fear of devascularizing the flaps during the operation. The increase in popularity of deep plane facelifts led to the concept of simultaneously applying chemical peels to the thicker facelift flaps. In 1994, Dingman and colleagues[23] studied phenol and TCA peels at various concentrations on skin flaps of pigs. The investigators then clinically performed 35% TCA peels on sub-SMAS facelift flaps and proved that TCA peel can safely be combined simultaneously with facelifts. However, they upheld Baker's original warning against combining a phenol peel simultaneously with facelift flaps. Despite the emergence of newer resurfacing technologies, some surgeons still prefer the reliability of chemical peels in combination with facelifts. Ozturk and colleagues[24] studied the outcomes of facelift combined with perioral phenol-croton oil peels and demonstrated patient satisfaction, objective evaluation of wrinkle improvement, and significant reduction in apparent age.

Laser Resurfacing

Laser resurfacing involves the application of heat energy in the form of photons to target a specific chromophore in the skin. The photons are *coherent* (in phase spatially and temporally in the form of waves with coinciding peaks and valleys) and *collimated* (do not spread out widely).[25]

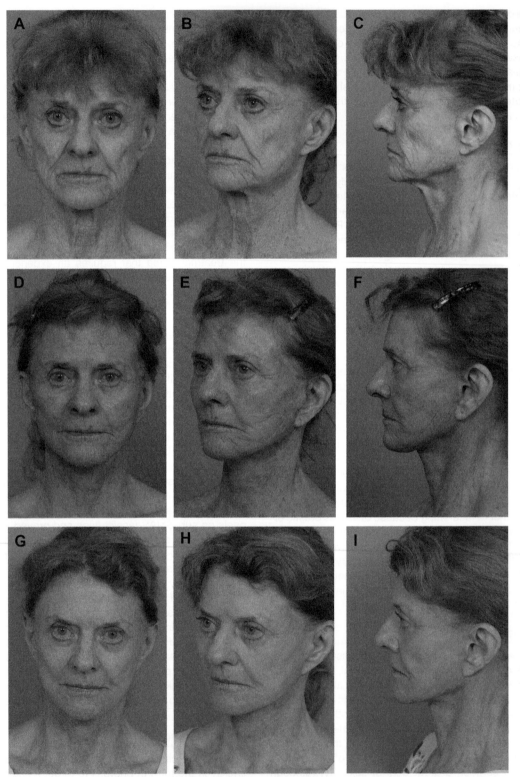

Fig. 1. An 80-year-old woman who underwent a facelift with fat grafting, full-face continuous ablative Er:YAG 2940-nm laser plus IPL, and botulinum toxin injection to the forehead and glabella. (*A–C*) Preoperative. (*D–F*) Twenty-five days postoperative immediately before laser plus IPL. (*G–I*) Four months postoperative and after nonsurgical adjuncts.

Hemoglobin, water, and melanin are examples of chromophores that are targeted in tissue. Each laser emits a *single (monochromatic)* wavelength that controls the depth of penetration and absorption by the intended chromophore. Lasers can be categorized as ablative versus nonablative and continuous (full-field) versus fractional.[26]

Ablative lasers apply thermal injury to both the epidermis and the dermis. *Nonablative* lasers treat the underlying dermis while preserving the overlying epidermis to minimize downtime and recovery. Therefore, the goal of a nonablative laser for aging is to stimulate neocollagenesis without creating a skin wound. Nonablative lasers include those in the midinfrared region, such as the 1064-nm Nd:YAG, and visible region, such as the pulsed dye laser (585–600 nm) and 532-nm potassium titanyl phosphate (KTP) laser. The pulsed dye laser and KTP lasers target hemoglobin as a chromophore. Therefore, these lasers are effective at treating vascular lesions, such as telangiectasias, and other red spots on the skin in facial rejuvenation patients.

Fractional lasers involve applying thermal energy to only a fraction (15%–25%) of the treated skin surface area in the form of regular arrays of narrow-diameter cylindrical columns separated by intervening areas of untreated skin. Fractional lasers are conventionally ablative. The intervening untreated skin allows the treated areas to be more rapidly repopulated with skin cells across the narrow column diameter rather than the single wide diameter of a continuous treatment area. The development of fractional lasers has been paramount in shortening recovery times (typically only a few days) with fewer side effects (discomfort, erythema, edema), but the results are not as impressive as with continuous lasers. Therefore, multiple treatment sessions (5–6) spaced at 1- to 4-week intervals are typically required. *Continuous* ablative lasers have a longer recovery period of about 2 weeks but typically produce impressive results after only a single treatment.

Carbon dioxide (CO_2) and erbium-doped yttrium aluminum garnet (Er:YAG) lasers target water as the chromophore in the skin and are considered the gold standard for resurfacing aged skin. The water in the tissue becomes heated, leading to a controlled tissue destruction. The CO_2 laser emits a 10,600-nm wavelength and the Er:YAG laser emits a 2940-nm wavelength in the far infrared range. Therefore, CO_2 has a deeper penetration depth (20–30 μm) compared with Er:YAG (1–3 μm), so the CO_2 laser causes greater tissue destruction. However, the depth of penetration can be increased by increasing the number of passes of the laser. The wavelength of the Er:YAG laser is close to the absorption peak of water, so it yields an absorption coefficient that is 16 times that of the CO_2 laser, leading to a more precise energy absorption and subsequent tissue destruction. This greater precision translates to less thermal injury to the surrounding skin and fewer side effects with shorter healing times. Considering the more precise absorption as a tradeoff for less depth of penetration and peripheral involvement, the Er:YAG has been associated with less tightening compared with the CO_2 laser, but the overall efficacy is considered similar. Both CO_2 and Er:YAG lasers are available in continuous and fractional capacities, and they are both effective at treating dyschromias in the form of brown spots in addition to rhytids.[26]

The use of lasers for facial rejuvenation emerged in the 1990s, beginning with the CO_2 laser. In 1997, Stuzin and colleagues[27] studied the histologic effects of CO_2 laser on photo-aged facial skin. The investigators performed laser resurfacing of the preauricular region in photo-damaged Caucasian patients before a facelift and compared the histologic findings of the laser-resurfaced test spots with the surrounding untreated photo-damaged skin. They found that the laser sites were clinically reepithelialized within 7 to 10 days; the epidermal atrophy and atypia were eliminated, and melanocytic hypertrophy and hyperplasia were corrected compared with the untreated photo-damaged skin. The histologic responses were also studied in African American patients and found to be similar to the Caucasian patients. In 1998, Guyuron and colleagues[28] reported delayed reepithelialization of skin flaps treated with CO_2 laser compared with skin flaps not treated with laser in a porcine model, and they reported delayed healing in 6 of 7 patients who underwent concomitant facelift and laser resurfacing. Later that year, Fulton demonstrated the safety of simultaneous TCA peel or short-pulse CO_2 laser with subcutaneous flaps and SMAS plication in 25 patients.[29] In 2000, Achauer and colleagues[30] reported a series of 26 patients who successfully underwent a sub-SMAS facelift with limited subcutaneous undermining and simultaneous full-face CO_2 laser resurfacing with lower fluence over the undermined skin, and discussion by Guyuron reported finding a laser energy level that is extremely safe when delivered simultaneously to the undermined skin. Since then, more articles have been published on the safety of combining facelift with laser resurfacing. The increased safety of combining facelift with laser resurfacing is also likely attributable to advances in laser technology with more types of lasers available and greater control of energy delivery. Moreira and colleagues[31] studied 80 patients who underwent subcutaneous facelift

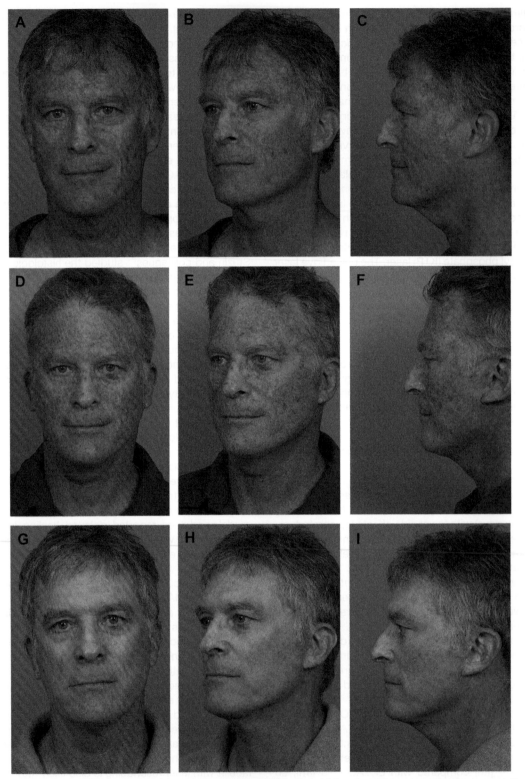

Fig. 2. A 66-year-old man who underwent a neck-lift, full-face hybrid fractional laser (nonablative coagulation 1470 nm and ablative vaporization 2940 nm) plus IPL, and botulinum toxin injection to the forehead, glabella, and crow's feet. (*A–C*) Preoperative. (*D–F*) Fourteen days postoperative immediately before laser plus IPL. (*G–I*) Five months postoperative and after nonsurgical adjuncts.

aps with SMAS plication and fractional laser resurfacing plus HA injection to the nasolabial folds and lips; they found a low incidence of major complications and high patient satisfaction. Scheuer and colleagues[32] reviewed 85 patients who underwent facelift with concomitant erbium laser resurfacing and reported a low rate of complications in the perioral, central, and full face.

Laser has the advantage of the extremely precise control of application by setting a specific wavelength, pulse duration, area of application, and energy (fluence) on the device. Lasers also possess a potential marketing advantage in patients who appeal to newer technologies. The main disadvantage of laser resurfacing is the high cost of each device and associated maintenance costs to the provider. Kitzmiller and colleagues[33] performed a split face study comparing a fractional CO_2 laser with dermabrasion of the perioral region and found that the laser had a significantly higher erythema score at 1 month and a small but significantly greater improvement in wrinkles at 6 months.

Laser resurfacing following a facelift is the preferred form of adjuvant facial resurfacing in the authors' practice. Facelift patients are assessed preoperatively for the severity of rhytids and photo-damage in addition to face/neck laxity. At the facelift consultation, patients with moderate or severe rhytids are offered laser resurfacing postoperatively as "icing on the cake" to maximize their facial rejuvenation. For those with *moderate* rhytids, the laser of choice in the authors' practice is a hybrid *fractional* laser that uses 2 wavelengths (nonablative coagulation with 1470 nm and ablative vaporization with 2940 nm). Utilization of dual wavelengths allows resurfacing at a more superficial and deeper depth, respectively, without extensive recovery (5–7 days). For those with *severe* rhytids, a *continuous* ablative 2940-nm laser is preferred for a more dramatic correction, which requires a longer recovery (10–14 days). Laser resurfacing can be performed in the early postoperative period to allow for 1 recovery, or may be performed in a delayed fashion at a later date. Early postoperative laser resurfacing is typically performed on the subcutaneous skin flaps at 1 to 2 weeks following a facelift. A single session is typically all that is needed postoperatively. Laser resurfacing does add considerable swelling to the surgical swelling, so the laser is not performed until the peak surgical swelling has started to subside at about a week. Patients with thin skin tend to have greater swelling, so laser resurfacing is typically delayed a little longer in the thinner-skinned patients and performed a little earlier in thicker-skinned patients. Avoiding additional swelling from the laser with concurrent peak surgical swelling is preferred to

prevent tension on the skin incisions during the first week. Facelift patients are typically advised that a 2-week recovery from bruising and swelling from surgery on the face is expected, and therefore, laser resurfacing performed during the early facelift recovery period does not substantially add recovery time, thus allowing for a single recovery period only. In addition, more aggressive laser resurfacing can theoretically be undertaken in the early postoperative period compared with immediately at the time of facelift after the vascularity to the skin flaps has had some time to improve. Laser resurfacing is also often combined with intense pulsed light (IPL) treatment of pigmentary lesions to maximize the adjuvant nonsurgical outcomes. **Figs. 1–3** demonstrate the results of patients who underwent laser resurfacing following facelift as well as other nonsurgical adjuncts.

Microneedling (Percutaneous Collagen Induction)

Although not truly considered skin resurfacing because the epidermis remains relatively intact, microneedling is a procedure that uses fine needles to puncture the skin, creating microwounds that stimulate release of growth factors and induce collagen production to improve the quality of the skin surface in a similar fashion.[34] Microneedling has also been combined with fractional radiofrequency to add a controlled thermal injury along with the mechanical injury of the microneedles to theoretically produce greater skin tightening.[35] Because it does not ablate the epidermis, microneedling is thought to avoid the risk of dyspigmentation present with the skin resurfacing modalities.[36] Therefore, microneedling may be a better option than resurfacing for nonsurgical skin rejuvenation in facelift patients with darker Fitzpatrick skin types (IV, V, VI).

INTENSE PULSED LIGHT

IPL is similar to laser resurfacing in that they both apply energy in the form of photons. However, light sources differ from lasers in that light sources produce *incoherent* light waves of *multiple* (*polychromatic*) wavelengths ranging from 550 to 1200 nm.[26] Filters are used to include or exclude certain wavelengths of IPL to treat only the intended targets. The intended chromophore is melanin and hemoglobin, so IPL is effective at treating brown and red spots. There can be a modest improvement of rhytids through release of heat energy into the dermis, resulting in neocollagenesis. However, the decrease in dyschromia and vascularity is much more impressive.[37]

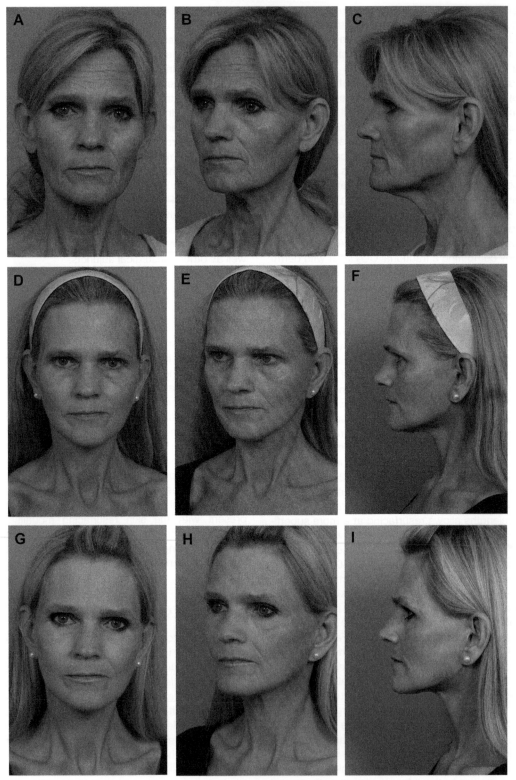

Fig. 3. A 54-year-old massive weight loss woman who underwent a facelift with fat grafting, full-face continuous ablative Er:YAG 2940-nm laser, and botulinum toxin injection to the forehead, glabella, crow's feet, and chin. (A–C) Preoperative. (D–F) Six weeks postoperative immediately before laser. (G–I) Four months postoperative and after nonsurgical adjuncts.

Recovery from an IPL treatment is minimal with 24 hours of slight erythema and edema.

NEUROMODULATORS

Botulinum toxin type A is a neuromodulator that blocks release of the neurotransmitter acetylcholine from the presynaptic axon at the neuromuscular junction, thereby inhibiting contraction of the target facial muscles and resultant conformational changes in the skin.[38] Richard Clark, a plastic surgeon from Sacramento, and Berris[39] were the first to document clinical use of botulinum toxin for cosmetic purposes. Clark used botulinum toxin to treat brow asymmetry caused by a unilateral frontal nerve injury during a facelift. Since then, the use of neuromodulators for purely aesthetic reasons has grown tremendously. Neuromodulators have since been used alone or as an adjunct to surgical procedures, such as a facelift to reduce forehead, glabellar, and lateral orbicularis (crow's feet) rhytids. They can also be used to reduce descent of the lateral oral commissure by blocking the depressor anguli oris (DAO) muscle, correction of excess gingival exposure (gummy smile), or platysmal bands. Some patients after a facelift may have incomplete correction of a descended lateral commissure with age and may benefit from the addition of botulinum toxin to the DAO postoperatively. Similarly, platysmal bands may be incompletely corrected or reappear following a lateral approach to the platysma or even a corset platysmaplasty, and these patients may benefit from botulinum toxin to the platysmal bands postoperatively. Therefore, botulinum toxin use following a facelift, brow-lift, or blepharoplasty should be considered synergistic rather than an alternative to surgery because these patients would benefit from continued botulinum toxin use postoperatively as part of life-long antiaging maintenance. Carruthers and Carruthers[40] studied the synergistic benefits of botulinum toxin combined with IPL compared with IPL alone and reported increased improvement with combined therapy.

SKIN CARE

For postoperative avoidance of further facial aging and sun damage following a facelift, a moisturizer with sun protection factor 30 sunscreen is recommended for daily use in the morning. At night, topical application of a retinoid is recommended. Retinoids have been shown to thin the outermost layer of the epidermis (stratum corneum) but thicken the granular layer with reversal of atypia, and they have been shown to increase neocollagenesis and angiogenesis and produce a more uniform dispersion of melanin granules in the dermis.[41] They also increase epidermal and dermal glycosaminoglycan deposition.[42] There is substantial evidence supporting the efficacy of prescription-grade retinoids (tretinoin, isotretinoin, alitretinoin); however, the evidence supporting less potent forms of retinoid-based cosmeceuticals (retinol, retinaldehyde, retinyl-palmitate, retinyl-acetate) is less well defined.[43] Large, randomized, controlled trials of cosmeceuticals containing retinaldehyde have been shown to have the most beneficial effect on aging skin.[44] Following laser resurfacing, a topical tripeptide/hexapeptide cream is recommended in the authors' practice to stimulate neoelastogenesis and neocollagenesis. A randomized, single-blinded trial of a tripeptide/hexapeptide healing regimen compared with a dimethicone-based ointment and petrolatum-based cream following laser resurfacing of the face reported improved outcomes in the tripeptide/hexapeptide group.[45]

SUMMARY

A facelift is effective at tightening laxity in the underlying support structures of the face/neck and removing the redundancy from aged facial skin, but patients also often exhibit other concomitant signs of facial aging that surgery does not address. By integrating the nonsurgical treatments outlined, plastic surgeons treating patients seeking facial rejuvenation can achieve optimal aesthetic outcomes beyond that which can be achieved with a facelift alone. At the time of consultation, patients should be assessed for signs of facial aging that can be treated with volume enhancement, skin resurfacing, IPL, neuromodulators, and skin care so that these nonsurgical options can be incorporated postoperatively to greatly enhance the outcomes of a facelift.

REFERENCES

1. Markarian MK, Hovsepian RV. The interface of cosmetic medicine and surgery: working from the inside and the outside. Clin Plast Surg 2011;38: 335–45.
2. Derby B, Codner MA. Evidence-based medicine: face lift. Plast Reconstr Surg 2017;139:151e–67e.
3. Marten TJ, Elyassnia D. Fat grafting in facial rejuvenation. Clin Plast Surg 2015;42:219–52.
4. Rohrich RJ, Ghavami A, Constantine FC, et al. Lift-and-fill face lift: integrating the fat compartments. Plast Reconstr Surg 2014;133:756e–67e.

5. Hammoudeh ZS, Small K, Unger JG, et al. Ear lobule rejuvenation in face-lifting: the role of fat augmentation. Plast Reconstr Surg Glob Open 2016;4:e597.

6. Wilson AJ, Taglienti AJ, Chang CS, et al. Current applications of facial volumization with fillers. Plast Reconstr Surg 2016;137:872e–89e.

7. Jones D. Volumizing the face with soft tissue fillers. Clin Plast Surg 2011;38:379–90.

8. Davidson BA. Lip augmentation using the palmaris longus tendon. Plast Reconstr Surg 1995;95:108–10.

9. Trussler AP, Kawamoto HK, Wasson KL, et al. Upper lip augmentation: palmaris longus tendon as an autologous filler. Plast Reconstr Surg 2008;121:1024–32.

10. Leaf N, Firouz JS. Lip augmentation with superficial musculoaponeurotic system grafts: report of 103 cases. Plast Reconstr Surg 2002;109:319–26.

11. Anderson RD. Alloplastic lip enhancement. Aesthet Surg J 2001;212:445–9.

12. Narsete T, Ersek R, Narsete MP. Further experience with permafacial implants for lip augmentation: a review of 100 implants. Aesthet Surg J 2011;31:488–92.

13. Lee DE, Hur SW, Lee JH, et al. Central lip lift as aesthetic and physiognomic plastic surgery: the effect on lower facial profile. Aesthet Surg J 2015;35:698–707.

14. Sherman RN. Sculptra: the new three-dimensional filler. Clin Plast Surg 2006;33:539–50.

15. Terino EO. Alloplastic facial contouring by zonal principles of skeletal anatomy. Clin Plast Surg 1992;19:487–510.

16. Smith JE. Dermabrasion. Facial Plast Surg 2014;30:35–9.

17. Alkhavam L, Alam M. Dermabrasion and microdermabrasion. Facial Plast Surg 2009;25:301–10.

18. Weissler JM, Carney MJ, Carreras Tartak JA, et al. The evolution of chemical peeling and modern-day applications. Plast Reconstr Surg 2017;140:920–9.

19. Hetter GP. An examination of the phenol-croton oil peel: part IV. Face peel results with different concentrations of phenol and croton oil. Plast Reconstructive Surg 2000;105:1061–83; discussion 1084–7.

20. Bensimon RH. Croton oil peels. Aesthet Surg J 2008;28:33–45.

21. Herbig K, Trussler AP, Khosla RK, et al. Combination Jessner's solution and trichloroacetic acid chemical peel: technique and outcomes. Plast Reconstr Surg 2009;124:955–64.

22. Baker TJ. Chemical face peeling and rhytidectomy. A combined approach for facial rejuvenation. Plast Reconstr Surg Transplant Bull 1962;29:199–207.

23. Dingman DL, Hartog J, Siemionow M. Simultaneous deep-plane face lift and trichloroacetic acid peel. Plast Reconstr Surg 1994;93:86–93 [discussion: 94–5].

24. Ozturk CN, Huettner F, Ozturk C, et al. Outcomes assessment of combination face lift and perioral phenol-croton oil peel. Plast Reconstr Surg 2013;132:743e–53e.

25. Gregory RO. Laser physics and physiology. Clin Plast Surg 1998;25:89–93.

26. Alexiades-Armenakas MR, Dover JS, Arndt KA. The spectrum of laser skin resurfacing: nonablative, fractional, and ablative laser resurfacing. J Am Acad Dermatol 2008;58:719–37.

27. Stuzin JM, Baker TJ, Baker TM, et al. Histologic effects of the high-energy pulsed CO_2 laser on photoaged facial skin. Plast Reconstr Surg 1997;99:2036–50.

28. Guyuron B, Michelow B, Schmelzer R, et al. Delayed healing of rhytidectomy flap resurfaced with CO2 laser. Plast Reconstr Surg 1998;101:816–9.

29. Fulton JE. Simultaneous face lifting and skin resurfacing. Plast Reconstr Surg 1998;102:2480–9.

30. Achauer BM, Adair SR, VanderKam VM. Combined rhytidectomy and full-face laser resurfacing. Plast Reconstr Surg 2000;106:1608–11 [discussion: 1612–3].

31. Moreira AC, Moreira M, Motta RL, et al. The combination of rhytidoplasty and fractional CO2 laser therapy in the treatment of facial aging. Aesthetic Plast Surg 2014;38:839–48.

32. Scheuer JF 3rd, Costa CR, Dauwe PB, et al. Laser resurfacing at the time of rhytidectomy. Plast Reconstr Surg 2015;136:27–38.

33. Kitzmiller WJ, Visscher M, Page DA, et al. The controlled evaluation of dermabrasion versus CO2 laser resurfacing for the treatment of perioral wrinkles. Plast Reconstr Surg 2000;106:1366–72.

34. Aust MC, Fernandes D, Kolokythas P, et al. Percutaneous collagen induction therapy: an alternative treatment for scars, wrinkles, and skin laxity. Plast Reconstr Surg 2008;121:1421–9.

35. Hou A, Cohen B, Haimovic A, et al. Microneedling: a comprehensive review. Dermatol Surg 2017;43:321–39.

36. Aust MC, Reimers K, Repenning C, et al. Percutaneous collagen induction: minimally invasive skin rejuvenation without risk of hyperpigmentation-fact or fiction? Plast Reconstr Surg 2008;122:1553–63.

37. Fodor I, Peled IJ, Rissin Y, et al. Using intense pulsed light for cosmetic purposes: our experience. Plast Reconstr Surg 2004;113:1789–95.

38. Noland ME, Lalonde DH, Yee GJ, et al. Current uses of botulinum neurotoxins in plastic surgery. Plast Reconstr Surg 2016;138:519e–30e.

39. Clark RP, Berris CE. Botulinum toxin: a treatment for facial asymmetry caused by facial nerve paralysis. Plast Reconstr Surg 1989;84:353–5.

0. Carruthers J, Carruthers A. The effect of full-face broadband light treatments alone and in combination with bilateral crow's feet botulinum toxin type A chemodenervation. Dermatol Surg 2004;30:355–66 [discussion 366].

1. Clark CP 3rd. Office-based skin care and superficial peels: the scientific rationale. Plast Reconstr Surg 1999;104:854–64.

2. Hubbard BA, Unger JG, Rohrich RJ. Reversal of skin aging with topical retinoids. Plast Reconstr Surg 2014;133:481e–90e.

43. Huang CK, Miller TA. The truth about over-the-counter topical anti-aging products: a comprehensive review. Aesthet Surg J 2007;27:402–12.

44. Babamiri K, Nassab R. Cosmeceuticals: the evidence behind the retinoids. Aesthet Surg J 2010; 30:74–7.

45. Vanaman Wilson MJ, Bolton J, Fabi SG. A randomized, single-blinded trial of a tripeptide/hexapeptide healing regimen following laser resurfacing of the face. J Cosmet Dermatol 2017;16: 217–22.

Perioperative Management of the Facelift Patient

Katherine B. Santosa, MD, MS[a], Jeremie D. Oliver, BS, BA[b],
Gina Thompson, BA[c], Richard J. Beil, MD[d,e,*]

KEYWORDS

- Aesthetics • Rhytidectomy • Preoperative care • Skin aging • Facial nerve • Hematoma
- Postoperative

KEY POINTS

- Perioperative management of the facelift patient is as important as the operation itself. It begins with understanding the process of aging on all the facial tissues and ends with a satisfied patient who has experienced no complications and has realized their desired result.
- Preoperative management needs to assess the patient's state of health and their expectations for the operation and prepare the patient to successfully undergo an operation.
- Postoperative care is designed to manage the physical and emotional needs of the patient to minimize complications and to ensure a successful outcome.

INTRODUCTION

Regardless of the technique of facelift chosen, there are universally important considerations for safe perioperative management of any patient undergoing a facelift. Understanding the physiologic and anatomic changes that occur with age and applying them to a comprehensive evaluation are skills critical to a successful preoperative consultation. Before surgery, it is also imperative to review the patient's comorbidities, medications, psychosocial well-being, and motivations for undergoing a facelift. The authors briefly review the concepts of informed consent and shared decision making, which can improve communication between the surgeon and patient and potentially reduce the risk of litigation. Before surgery, the anesthetic plan should be outlined and tailored to the individual patient. Postoperative pain management drains and dressings and skin care are also discussed. Vigilance to perioperative management of a facelift patient is important to ensuring the safety of the patient, facilitating an uneventful recovery period with heightened patient satisfaction.

PREOPERATIVE CONSIDERATIONS
Changes in the Face with Aging

Understanding how different components of the face are altered with aging is essential to effectively evaluating any patient interested in undergoing a facelift. In this section, the authors review the anatomic and physiologic changes that occur to the face with aging.

Skin changes

Skin alterations with aging are a result of both intrinsic and extrinsic factors. Inevitably,

Disclosure Statement: The authors have nothing to disclose.
[a] Section of Plastic Surgery, Department of Surgery, University of Michigan, 1500 East Medical Center Drive, Ann Arbor, MI 48109, USA; [b] Mayo Clinic School of Medicine, 200 First Street Southwest, Rochester, MN 55905, USA; [c] Pierre Fabre USA, 8 Campus Drive, 2nd Floor, Parsippany, NJ 07054, USA; [d] Center for Plastic and Reconstructive Surgery, 5333 McAuley Drive, Suite 5001, Ypsilanti, MI 48197, USA; [e] University of Michigan, Ann Arbor, MI, USA
* Corresponding author. Center for Plastic and Reconstructive Surgery, 5333 McAuley Drive, Suite 5001, Ypsilanti, MI 48197, USA.
E-mail address: Rjbeilmd8@gmail.com

https://doi.org/10.1016/j.cps.2019.06.008
0094-1298/19/

chronologic aging is genetically influenced, leading to cutaneous rhytids and laxity. Extrinsically linked factors influencing facial skin aging include environmental toxins, gravity, and most importantly, UV sun exposure.[1] Histology of the aging skin demonstrates a constellation of findings, including (1) thinning of the epidermis, (2) flattening of the rete ridges at the dermal-epidermal junction, (3) thinning and degeneration of the reticular and papillary layers of the dermis, collagen bundles, and elastic fibers, as well as (4) atrophy of subcutaneous tissue.[2] In addition, skin atrophy and laxity are affected by a decrease in cellular turnover and collagen synthesis.[3] Further clinical signs of extrinsic effects on aging skin include dryness, pigment irregularity, loss of elasticity, telangiectasias, and areas of purpura.[1]

Soft tissue changes

As a consequence of the aging process, the once youthful appearance of the face becomes attenuated by volumetric and ligamentous changes in the soft tissue structure. Laxity of facial skin relative to the retaining ligaments combined with fat redistribution anteriorly and inferiorly in the malar region produces a square shape to the once tapered and full midface.[4] As facial fat is situated caudally, the appearance of the face becomes elongated vertically in a gradual overall descent of soft tissue structural support. Regions more densely populated by retaining ligaments in the face tend to be most severely impacted by fat deflation and volume loss with aging (eg, nasolabial folds and marionette lines).[5] Volumetric deflation with age occurs in the following regions: malar, preparotid, infraorbital and lateral orbital rim, and pogonion, most notably at the mobile anterior aspect of the face, with subsequent age-related changes in the lateral aspects where superficial and deep layers are strongly adherent to each other.[6] As a result, previously smooth transitions between youthful aesthetic subunits of the face, particularly along the nasolabial fold and mandibular angle, become demarcated with fat deflation and descent.[7] Importantly, however, the aging effects on the face are not limited to vertical descent of soft tissue.[4] Radial expansion of facial soft tissue is particularly noted in the midface, thought to be attributed as an effect of prolonged animation and radial motion of smiling, which weakens the facial musculature and fascial support. This anatomical change accounts for prominence of the nasolabial fold noted in the aging face, as skin and subcutaneous soft tissue structures expand radially following prolonged lateral motion stress over time, thus causing a prolapse from underlying facial skeletal insertion.[4] A similar effect is seen lateral to the oral commissure

along the marionette lines, accounting for some of the consequential jowling from radial expansion as superficial soft tissue structures lose their adhesion to the deep fascial support of the face.[5] Structures contributing to jowling with age include the mandibular septum, separating jowl from neck fat, traveling across and adhering to the anterior surface of the body of the mandible, as well as the mandibular septum, which tethers skin to the border of the mandible similar to the temporal septa and cheek septa, further suggesting that facial rejuvenation is optimized when surgical approaches are performed in a site-specific manner.[8]

Facial skeletal changes

As in all bony structures of the aging human body, the facial skeleton experiences age-related loss of mass and mineral density, with accompanied increase in marrow fat content and altered hormonal responsiveness.[9] This degenerative process is juxtaposed by a progressive expansion of facial skeletal features, evident in certain facial anthropometric measurements, such as nasion-to-anterior nasal spine and overall facial width.[10,11] As these 2 competing processes of bone resorption along with bone deposition coincide in the aging facial skeleton, the orbital aperture increases in both area and width,[12] contributing to the "sunken-in" appearance of the periorbital region. Earlier manifestations of facial aging occur along the inferolateral orbital rim (by middle age), whereas superomedial or inferomedial quadrant periorbital bony changes become more evident with increasing age.[13,14] In addition, midface fullness decreases with age, on average by about 10° from age 30 to age 60.[14] Nasal bone morphology is also altered with age, characterized by lengthening of the nose, tip droop, and posterior displacement of the columella and lateral crurae.[15] Further clinical manifestation of bony change around the nasal structure includes posterior displacement of the alar base relative to the medial canthi, indicating bony loss in the lower pyriform aperture, often presenting with deepening of the nasolabial fold.[16,17] Likely as a result of these bony changes, superimposed by soft tissue descent with the forces of gravity, the lower half of the face has been shown to expand continuously with aging.[18,19] The formation of jowls in the aging lower face is thought to often be a result of reduced skeletal projection at the prejowl sulcus region, leading to development of a relative concavity, such as in younger patients with congenital microgenia.[18,20]

Contribution of these different changes leads to the appearance of the aging face; however, it is important to note that only some of these factors can be adequately addressed by an operation.

Often, in patients with severe facial rhytids, especially those from sun exposure, resurfacing techniques should be implemented as part of the rejuvenation plan.

Initial Consultation and Analysis of the Face

Preoperative evaluation of the patient's face involves inspection and palpation of facial structures. In determining the ideal treatment strategies for the patient seeking facial rejuvenation, consideration of the individual patient's objective facial structure and aesthetics based on systematic mapping (ie, splitting the face into thirds: upper, mid, and lower face) and 3-dimensional evaluation of all structures of the face provide insight as to the best techniques to use. One such approach may be to use a top-down analysis of facial composition and symmetry or lack thereof.[21] Assessment of the patient's Fitzpatrick skin type, overall facial fat content, and facial asymmetry is of particular importance, because patients with higher Fitzpatrick skin types may have a tendency for hypertrophic scar formation and pigmentation changes along incision lines.[22] Patients presenting with less baseline volume as a result of more advanced aging tend to demonstrate better postoperative contour improvement when compared with patients with greater facial soft tissue volume.[14] Most patients present with at least some degree of facial asymmetry, often originating at the level of the bony skeleton.[14] Addressing each of these objective findings on initial consultation is an important step in discussing treatment options with the patient as well as a necessary measure to help buffer postoperative expectations (see preoperative photographs; **Figs. 1**A-B, **2**A-B).

At the completion of the initial evaluation, diagnoses and findings from examination are discussed openly with the patient. This discussion should encompass and emphasize the patient's initial expressed concerns as well as any additional findings noted by the surgeon. Going through this formal evaluation process allows the surgeon to gain a better sense of the patient's perception of his or her facial features and the desires for rejuvenation, thus allowing the surgeon to individualize treatment plans and recommendations on a patient-specific level.

To a certain extent, there is a physician bias brought to bear on every consultation. It stems from the surgeon's philosophic approach to the facelift patient, which likely is influenced by experience and may change with time. Some physicians want to stress the improvement that can be achieved in offering (and in some cases insisting) that the patient have the entire face, brow,

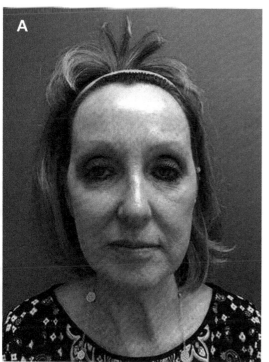
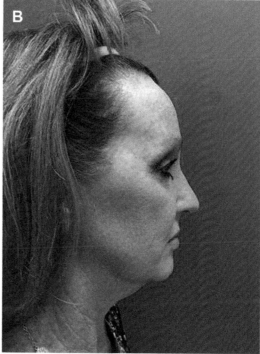

Fig. 1. Preoperative consult for patient 1. (*A*) Anteroposterior view. (*B*) Right lateral view.

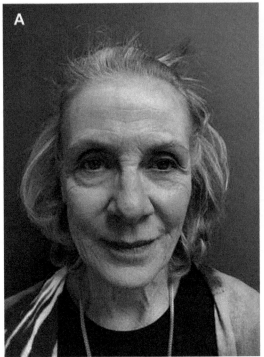 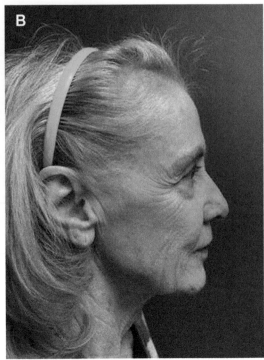

Fig. 2. Preoperative consult for patient 2. (*A*) Anteroposterior view. (*B*) Right lateral view.

eyelids, and neck be addressed simultaneously. For other physicians, a more patient-centered focus of operations to be performed is preferred, as long as changes created by the planned operations that could influence adjacent areas to the face are noted.

Adjunctive procedures, such as brow-lift surgery, blepharoplasty, autologous fat transfer, and facial resurfacing, in conjunction with facelift surgery, which may enhance the final outcome, should be brought to the patient's attention.[23,24] Previous facelift patients' preoperative and postoperative photographs may be useful in demonstrating the intended benefits of proposed treatments. A keen level of sensitivity toward the patient's desires is essential. In many cases, gentle guidance from the surgeon can facilitate patients' recognition of the added benefits of adjunctive procedures, when indicated.[25] Caution should certainly be practiced in patients who are unreasonably resistant to the surgeon's clinical impression, because such behavior may indicate potential postoperative noncompliance and higher risk for compromised surgical outcomes. If the surgeon feels like their ability to connect with the patient is lacking at any point during the consultation, the surgeon may want to dissuade the patient from having surgery with them and encourage a second

opinion, or simply decline to operate on the patient. This decision will reduce potential difficulties for both the patient and the physician in the future.

Informed Consent and Shared Decision Making

Maintaining realistic expectations is essential to optimize patient satisfaction postoperatively. Full transparency with patient education in mind during the preoperative consultation allows for a more realistic understanding of the potential risks and benefits of undergoing facial aesthetic surgery and will help the surgeon optimize patient safety and satisfaction. During the initial consultation, a clear outline of the postoperative limitations/restrictions should be detailed to allow for the patient to decide if and when the procedure will fit into their daily life routine.

Informed consent is necessary to facilitate effective communication between the surgeon and patient.[26] The surgeon has the responsibility of fully disclosing potential risks and complications, benefits, and alternatives of undergoing a facelift, within the proper context and with relative incidence rates. An important component of the informed consent process for the facelift operation is the discussion regarding management of potential complications. Given the elective nature of facelift surgery, complications such as hematoma or nerve injury, which could require additional surgical intervention and/or additional testing, may not be covered by insurance. In these situations, patients may have to pay out of pocket for management of complications if they do not elect to obtain insurance through one of the cosmetic insurance plans designed specifically for these incidences. After a surgeon has fully disclosed risks, benefits, and potential alternatives of a procedure, patients have the opportunity to provide consent or refuse.[27] Among facial and plastic surgery procedures, repeated studies have demonstrated that litigation and malpractice claims are less likely due to technical faults, but more attributed to lack of informed consent and inadequate and poor communication between the surgeon and patient.[26,28,29] For example, a recent study found that 34% of malpractice litigation cases after facelift were attributed to inadequate informed consent.[30]

Because patients desire greater participation in health care decisions, there has been an effort over the past several decades to go beyond informed consent toward the adoption of shared decision making (SDM), especially in elective procedures.[31] SDM is a collaborative process by which the patient and physician come to a mutually agreed upon, appropriate treatment plan that aligns with the patient's values, preferences, and circumstance[32-34] and is especially important in situations in which multiple options exist, such as those in aesthetic surgery.[35] Using decision aids to promote SDM not only reduces risk of litigation among facelift patients[36] but also can improve patients' knowledge of different treatment options, such as location of incision and technique of facelift. Although many providers believe they are already engaging in SDM during the informed consent process by explaining the procedure, its risks, benefits, and potential alternatives, this 1-way mode of communication does not elicit the patient's preference, differentiating it from SDM.[35] Using SDM, patients report improved satisfaction and are more compliant with their chosen treatment plan, emphasizing the positive impact of SDM on consultations with patients undergoing elective procedures such as facelift.[37,38]

Preoperative Medical Management

The typical elective aesthetic surgery patient tends to be relatively healthy. Interestingly, older age does not confer an increased risk of complications.[39] However, among patients with comorbidities, regardless of age, the plastic surgeon should obtain preoperative clearance from the patient's primary care physician or an internal medicine specialist to help manage any chronic diseases and weigh the benefits against the potential risks of surgery in the setting of these medical comorbidities. Patients with severe systemic diseases, such as heart failure, renal failure, and poorly controlled diabetes, are not candidates for a facelift. Poor glycemic control places diabetic patients seeking *any* aesthetic surgery procedure at increased risk of surgical site infection and delayed wound healing.[40] Certain disorders of the skin, including Ehlers-Danlos syndrome, progeria, and elastoderma, are associated with severe wound healing difficulty; thus, surgery in individuals with these disorders is contraindicated.[2] In contrast, individuals with loose skin, such as in conditions like cutis laxa or pseudoxanthoma elasticum, may benefit from facial aesthetic surgery.[41]

There is no debate that cigarette smoking has a negative effect on the process of wound healing by way of driving tissue hypoxia and ischemia,[42] because smokers have a 12 times increase in complications than non-smokers undergoing a facelift.[43] In the event that a patient who is a current smoker presents for consultation, common practice is to enforce a 4- to 6-week time period before and after the operation in which the patient does not smoke.[44] In order to promote absolute compliance, it may be in the patient's and surgeon's best interest to facilitate pharmacologic (ie, varenicline, bupropion prescription) and nonpharmacologic (ie, counseling, cognitive behavior therapy, electrical stimulation, etc.) interventions in order to achieve smoking abstinence and perhaps cessation. Among smokers who quit before the operation, surgeons may elect to perform different facelift techniques (ie, deep plane vs dual plane) to potentially decrease the risk of skin loss in these higher-risk patients. Although 4 to 6 weeks of abstinence may be the minimum requested for some, clearly a longer period of nicotine-free living before an operation is safer for the patient to avoid the complications of skin loss associated with this practice. Having the patient be nicotine free for 6 months is not unreasonable given the magnitude of the potential complication.

Medication Review

Before undergoing a facelift, every patient's current medication list should be carefully reviewed by the plastic surgeon and adjusted, if necessary, to decrease the risks of bleeding, adverse interactions with anesthetic medications, and hypercoagulability. Although complications following a facelift have been studied exhaustively over the past several decades, factors shown to consistently predispose patients to complications include preoperative intake of aspirin or other antiplatelet drugs, active smoking, intraoperative use of epinephrine, postoperative vomiting, and poorly controlled blood pressure.[45–50]

An important component of the medication list in a patient seeking aesthetic facial surgery is any herbal supplements the patient may be taking, because several these have been cited for adverse reactions during or after surgery.[51] As such, the surgeon should instruct the patient to abstain from all herbal supplements at least 2 to 3 weeks before the date of the operation (recommendation by the American Society of Anesthesiologists).[52] Some of these herbal remedies include chondroitin (bleeding risk), Echinacea (barbiturate and halothane toxicity, allergic reaction, immunotoxicity), ephedra (cardiac effects), garlic (bleeding), gingko (bleeding), glucosamine (hypoglycemia), goldenseal (photosensitivity, sedation), kava root (sedation), and milk thistle (volume depletion).[52] In addition, some common foods have been linked to increased risk of postoperative bleeding. Surgeons may advise their patients to abstain from these foods for a period of 1 to 2 weeks before and after surgery: avocado, apple, cucumber, fish (salmon, in particular), garlic, grapefruit, grapes, lemons, oranges, raspberries, strawberries, soybeans, sweet potatoes, and wheat germ oil, among others.[2] Providing lists of prescription medications, over-the-counter supplements, and foods to avoid can be very helpful to the patient.

Considerations of Anesthesia

Anesthetic technique has a tremendous effect on appropriate control of blood pressure, anxiety, pain, and nausea and is essential for reducing the facelift hematoma risk.[53] Despite the fact that the facelift procedure can successfully be performed under intravenous sedation or general anesthesia, basic tenets of adequate hemodynamic monitoring and control apply universally regardless of anesthetic approach. In the interest of blood pressure control, this can be optimized by controlling influential stressors, including pain, anxiety, nausea, and vomiting. An appropriate preoperative, intraoperative, and postoperative medication regimen can minimize the risk of patients developing hematoma postoperatively. Intraoperatively, blood pressure should be maintained normotensive throughout the case.[53] If performing

the operation under general anesthesia, at the time of induction and airway manipulation, a combination of propofol, inhalational agents, and neuromuscular blockade allows for a smooth transition with minimal airway irritation and stable vital signs.[54]

There are some medications that can improve patients' experience and facilitate a smoother recovery. For example, benzodiazepines are an effective option in the immediate preoperative setting to reduce anxiety.[53] Postoperative nausea and vomiting may be reduced or diminished by administering antiemetics before or shortly following induction and/or before emergence.[55] Optimal blood pressure may be maintained not only by controlling emesis and pain but also with the addition of a clonidine transdermal patch, placed preoperatively especially in the patient with marginal blood pressure control.[56] This preoperative intervention should always be done with the knowledge and consent of the primary care provider.

Overall, the facelift procedure is safe, well tolerated, and very amenable to standard anesthetic protocols for successful outcomes. Likely the most worrisome potential complication in regards to maintenance anesthesia before, during, and following the operation is inadequate blood pressure control. Measures should be established between the operating plastic surgeon and anesthesia care provider in order to prevent this readily treatable risk factor,[57] emphasizing the importance of close communication with the anesthesia team in order to facilitate a safe and successful facelift operation.

Skin Optimization Before Surgery

Preoperative skin care management of the facelift patient provides the opportunity to optimize skin health before the operation and introduce concepts of postoperative skin care management and camouflage makeup that will be useful after the operation. In the authors' practice, patients meet with an aesthetician specialized in skin care for a 1-hour consultation 4 to 6 weeks before surgery to create a customized preoperative skincare regimen and review instructions for postoperative skin management.

To optimize skin health before surgery, the authors prescribe a regimen that includes the following 5 steps (**Table 1**):

1. Cleanse;
2. Moisturize;
3. Exfoliate;
4. Protect;
5. Repair.

Table 1
Preoperative skincare regimen

1. Cleanse	Prescribe cleanser with antibacterial components (eg, glycolic acid) to remove dirt, debris, and oil. Prepares skin for subsequent steps in skincare regimen
2. Moisturize	Keeping the skin moist is important to maintaining a lipid barrier and more resilient epidermis
3. Exfoliate	Exfoliating agents (eg, vitamin A or alpha-hydroxy acids) facilitate cell turnover, which results in brighter, smoother skin
4. Protect	Protect the skin from sun exposure using products with SPF 30 or higher
5. Repair	Reparative ingredients may include aloe vera, vitamin C, vitamin E, coenzyme Q10, and green tea. These ingredients may increase hydration and improve elasticity

A cleanser with an antibacterial component, such as glycolic acid or plant-based essential oils, removes dirt, debris, and oil and prepares the skin for subsequent steps in the skincare regimen. Moisturization is essential to maintaining a healthy lipid barrier and more resilient epidermis.[58] Next, exfoliating agents, such as those with vitamin A or alpha hydroxy acids, facilitate cell turnover, which will not only contribute to a brighter, smoother, and more youthful-looking appearance but also create a more permeable skin surface for effective product absorption. Because exfoliating agents can be irritating to some skin types, it should not be used more than once a day, preferably at night, and should be monitored for tolerance. Protecting the skin during hours of sun exposure with products that contain a sun protection factor (SPF) of 30 or higher is a daily practice that can prevent photodamage and premature aging and maintain healthy skin. The authors believe that encouraging compliance of this practice preoperatively may ultimately help preserve the results of the operation. Reparative skin treatments are beneficial in addressing acute skin issues and also preventing long-term effects of aging. Ingredients such as aloe vera, vitamin C, vitamin E, coenzyme Q10, and green tea can provide reparative and protective benefits to damaged skin and may also improve elasticity, increase hydration levels, reduce redness and surface irritation, minimize acne lesions, and improve overall skin health.[2]

Psychosocial Evaluation

During the consultation, the surgeon should review the patient's mental health history and support system. Mental illness in our society is not uncommon, and patients presenting for cosmetic surgery are more likely to have a history of depression than the general population.[59,60] For patients with extensive psychiatric histories, such as previous hospitalization or the presence of psychotic disorders (eg, schizophrenia), it is important to obtain psychiatric clearance to ensure emotional stability of the surgical patient. In addition to assessing the patient's mental health history, an equally important consideration is the support system of the patient.

In addition, the surgeon should assess the patient's motivation for surgery. Commonly reported motivations include improving one's self-image and advancing one's career,[61] which are generally considered reasonable motives, but it is prudent to be especially thorough in the initial consultation process to uncover potential hidden agendas or unstated impetuses that may be less obvious or unrealistic. If a patient is excessively preoccupied with a nonexistent or very subtle flaw in their appearance,[62] they should be carefully screened for body dysmorphic disorder (BDD), because these individuals are poor candidates for aesthetic surgery.[63] A recent study suggests that about 13% of patients undergoing aesthetic surgery had BDD,[64] but that surgeons only correctly identify BDD in 4.7% of all patients.[65] If BDD is suspected in a patient, the surgeon should refer them to a psychiatrist for further management.[63,64]

POSTOPERATIVE CARE
Drains, Dressings, and Postoperative Restrictions

Drains can be used during a facelift procedure. Timing of when to remove the drains is at the surgeon's discretion. Anecdotally in the authors' experience, leaving a drain in for a few days postoperatively has resulted in fewer complications compared with drainless approaches. The authors loosely apply dressings not to prevent hematoma but to absorb any expected drainage from the incision sites. Use of compression after facelift surgery is controversial and should be used at the discretion of the surgeon's preference and experience. Some believe that compression after surgery can result in skin loss, whereas others use the compression to maintain surgical results and compress any dead space between skin flaps. The authors' preference is to loosely apply an ACE bandage circumferentially for 1 week.

In the authors' practice, they advise patients to avoid any heavy lifting of more than 10 pounds, bending at the waist, strenuous activity of any sort, and straining for 2 weeks after surgery. Patients can resume exercise slowly between the second and third weeks and then are unrestricted beginning the third week after surgery.

Preventing a Hematoma

Even with meticulous precautions preoperatively (ie, avoidance of platelet function inhibitors, adequate control of hypertension) and intraoperatively by achieving thorough hemostasis, hematoma incidence is to be expected at a minimum of 1% to 2%.[4] Despite this relatively high incidence, postoperative expanding hematoma can be properly controlled and managed when promptly recognized by the surgeon. Preoperative management of baseline hypertension is critical to decrease the risk of hematoma. Clonidine (0.3 mg) given approximately 1 hour preoperatively can be useful in achieving adequate low blood pressure during the perioperative period, in addition to any other medications for blood pressure modulation the patient may be taking. Intraoperatively, as well as in the immediate postoperative period, the anesthesiologist may administer blood pressure–lowering agents in the event that the patient's systolic reading increases to greater than 120 mm Hg.[66]

Male patients in particular carry a much higher risk of postoperative hematoma following rhytidectomy given the highly vascular, sebaceous, thick facial skin compared with the female patient.[4] Extra precaution is warranted by way of preoperative blood pressure management and complete intraoperative hemostasis in the male patient facelift in order to optimize surgical outcomes.

Postoperative monitoring of the patient following facelift for any potential immediate complication is critical within the first 3 to 4 hours after the operation, because this is the period during which most expanding hematomas will manifest.[67] Associated symptoms of hematoma in this immediate postoperative period include pain, restlessness, nausea, and blood pressure elevation. Any patient reporting these symptoms within this postoperative timeframe should be closely monitored in order to maximize intervention effect.[68] Clinical signs to be aware of during monitoring of the patient for hematoma risk include hardness of the neck and/or cheek, eversion of the lips, and bluish discoloration of the buccal mucosa on the affected side.[4]

Early intervention in suspected expanding hematoma is the most reliable measure to prevent devastating complications of the facelift surgery such as airway compromise or necrosis of skin flaps. If possible, the patient should be brought back to the operating room should there be evidence of hematoma expansion for suture removal of the affected side and thorough inspection of area of concern beneath the flap.[66] The wound should be sufficiently irrigated with normal saline and all clots removed with sponged forceps before a reattempt at hemostasis and approximation of skin edges along flap incision.

Other Key Complications Following Facelift

Sensory nerve injury is the next most-common complication reported following facelift surgery with the great auricular nerve being most commonly damaged.[69] Estimated incidence of great auricular nerve injury during facelift is reported as high as 2.6%.[70] This nerve can be identified during cervical flap elevation from the sternocleidomastoid muscle fascia; should there be an inadvertent laceration of the nerve, primary repair under loupe magnification is performed with fine suture in an attempt to restore full sensory function of the nerve.[4] Importantly, most facelift patients report only transient sensory disturbances due to transection of smaller sensory nerves over the preauricular and anterior neck regions of skin flap elevation.

Motor nerve injury in rhytidectomy tends to be transient, with complete resolution by 3 to 4 months in most cases. The most commonly affected nerve is the buccal branch of the facial nerve; however, frontal, mandibular, and cervical branch weakness has also been reported, with an overall variable incidence likely less than 1%.[71] Neurologic signs of injury are present postoperatively based on the nerve branch affected. Most common routes of iatrogenic injury to the nerve branches include cautery trauma, suture placement within nerve track, or (most commonly) stretch-induced transient neuropraxia.[4] Patients should be counseled preoperatively as well as in the postoperative period in order to help them anticipate likely duration of symptoms.

Scarring is an inevitable consequence, regardless of meticulous surgical technique for optimal placement and excellent postoperative incision care. Some patients more than others will have a tendency to develop hypertrophic or undesirable scars over the subsequent postoperative months. Such scarring can be managed as needed with intralesional steroid injections, often relinquishing any additional intervention to manage the undesired scarring. Positive effects of direct injection of steroid into the scar tissue include atrophy of hypertrophic scar, reduction in erythema, pruritus, and pain as the incisions heal.[4] However, should intralesional steroid management prove insufficient for optimal scar reduction after 6 to 12 months postoperatively, additional operative excision of scar tissue can be performed.

Although a rare complication following rhytidectomy, superficial infection of the wound may occur in less than 1% of cases.[23] The most commonly implicated microbe associated with a facelift wound infection is *Staphylococcus aureus*.[4] Given the placement of pretragal incision near the external ear canal, perioperative antibiotics to minimize skin flora infection of the facelift flaps may be given (typically cephalosporin or vancomycin, coverage against *S aureus* and *Staphylococcus epidermidis*). The most common presenting sign of facelift wound infection is neck erythema, which can be quickly identified postoperatively and managed by oral antibiotic modulation to sufficiently cover possible inciting organisms. Should the infection go undetected in the initial postoperative period, the facial flap may become suppurative and require intravenous antibiotics along with operative incision and drainage and potential hyperbaric oxygen therapy to assure adequate wound healing.[4]

Likely the most severe complication reported following rhytidectomy is flap necrosis. The cause of such a devastating complication is likely multifactorial, with tissue ischemia, underlying skin infection, thin elevated flaps, and microvascular insufficiency (eg, patients with history of smoking) contributing on a case-by-case basis.[43] Furthermore, postoperative wound care becomes crucial in assuring appropriate (but not over tightly wrapped) dressings in order to minimize edema while avoiding constriction of blood flow. Should skin slough manifest, the wound should be left to heal by secondary intention. Allow for adequate granulation and reepithelialization before considering skin grafting or debridement.[4]

Pain Management

Ensuring patient comfort after elective aesthetic surgery is paramount to a successful surgical outcome. An important component of ensuring patient comfort is effective pain control in the acute postoperative period, which undoubtedly leads to improved patients outcomes and patient satisfaction.[72] Opioids are effective and remain the cornerstone in controlling acute postoperative pain; however, opioids may be harmful and should be prescribed judiciously. Long-term opioid use among facial aesthetic surgery patients has yet to be examined, but population-level analyses demonstrate that about 6% to 10% of patients who were previously opioid naïve before surgery become dependent on opioids after different types of plastic surgery procedures.[73,74] Screening for risk factors for new persistent opioid use, such as anxiety, depression, and history of alcohol and substance use disorders,[75] should be incorporated in the preoperative consultation so that an individualized pain management strategy can be outlined for these higher-risk patients. Another important consideration of opioid prescribing is concomitant use of benzodiazepines because this increases a patient's risk of emergency department visit, hospital admission for drug-related emergency, overdose, and even death.[76,77] Extreme caution in opioid prescribing should be taken among patients who use benzodiazepines.

Facelift patients should also be counseled on the potential unwanted side effects of opioid use, which include nausea, vomiting, sedation, dizziness, constipation, and urinary retention. Given these undesirable side effects, surgeons may consider prescribing adjuncts to opioids for acute postoperative pain. Intravenous acetaminophen may be considered in the immediate postoperative setting.[53] In addition, celecoxib, a cyclooxygenase-2 inhibitor, which lacks the adverse effects of antiplatelet function, has been shown to be effective in reducing pain and opioid consumption among patients undergoing facelift.[78] If opioids are prescribed for a rhytidectomy patient, the authors suggest the taking the following precautions:

1. Educate the patient about the adverse effects and risk for misuse and abuse of opioids even after short-term use of these medications.
2. Among patients who are opioid naïve before surgery, screen for risk factors of prolonged opioid use during preoperative visits. For patients who use opioids for chronic pain conditions before surgery, communicate with the patient's opioid prescriber (eg, primary care physician, pain specialist) regarding postoperative pain management and adhere to the 1-prescriber rule.
3. Use extreme caution and try to avoid prescribing opioids to a patient who is concomitantly taking a benzodiazepine.
4. Prescribe a short course of opioids (eg, 3 days) and closely reassess the patient's

postoperative pain levels at clinic visit to avoid overprescribing.

5. Encourage patients to dispose of any unused opioid medications and provide information regarding safe disposal techniques and take-back locations.

Postoperative Psychosocial Issues

Although emphasis is placed on psychosocial evaluation to rule out conditions like BDD and any "red-flag" motivations driving the desire for surgery preoperatively, recognizing and managing psychosocial issues of facelift patients postoperatively are equally as important. Men and women who undergo facial aesthetic surgery, such as facelifts, report significantly improved satisfaction and quality of life, highlighting the benefits of these procedures.[79,80] However, for a period of time after surgery, some patients may experience psychosocial and emotional distress before their quality of life is actually improved.[60,61]

Goin and colleagues[61] found that 54% of facelift patients had some sort of psychological disturbance after surgery. In addition, after evaluating these patients for 6 months postoperatively, they found that about 30% patients had depressive symptoms.[61] Although the cause of their psychological disturbances or depressive symptoms was not investigated in their study, the authors can speculate that, for some, negative feelings after surgery may be due to physical pain, discomfort, or unforeseen complications; however, they may also be attributed to the unsightly appearance of redness, bruising, and swelling that occurs in the immediate postoperative period leading to social isolation and/or deeper emotional feelings of guilt, shame, and regret. Unlike other aesthetic procedures of the body, physical side effects of a facelift or other facial aesthetic procedure can be difficult to hide and may result in a longer period of social isolation. For some patients, social and emotional support after surgery may be nonexistent, which could also contribute to the problem.[60,61]

Recognizing that many facelift patients may experience psychosocial distress after surgery is imperative for plastic surgeons to successfully manage these patients in the perioperative period. First, the authors suggest incorporating other members of the surgical team and practice, such as a massage therapist or aesthetician, into the routine postoperative course. Outside of follow-up visits with the surgeon, these visits with other team members provide other opportunities for patients to end their isolation in a supportive environment while also allowing them to voice their concerns whereby creating a more emotionally supportive postsurgical environment. Second, simple reassurances, by any team member, particularly during the first week of recovery, that reinforce that the patient will heal, discomfort will subside, bruises will fade, and a more "normal" appearance will be restored, that seem relatively obvious to the medical provider can be very helpful in reducing fear and anxiety. Third, the authors encourage providing facelift patients with a camouflage makeup lesson. During this session, patients learn how to safely apply a special makeup with superior coverage to areas that are red or bruised, in an effort to minimize social isolation. In the authors' experience, patients better appreciate the results of their operation immediately after they are able to conceal bruising and redness (see postoperative photographs; **Figs.** 3A-B, 4A-B).

Postoperative Skincare Regimen

Postoperative skin care management is an important component of the management of a patient who has undergone a facelift (**Table 2**). The authors define it as a 3-phase process, as follows:

1. Immediate skin care, which encompasses the first 7 to 14 days after surgery;
2. Interim skin care, 1 to 10 weeks after the operation;
3. Maintenance skin care, designed to maintain optimal skin health indefinitely.

During the immediate phase of postoperative skin care management, it is imperative that patients understand that they should not apply any topical agents to any open wounds or healing incisions unless specifically prescribed by their surgeon. Surgeons can recommend that their patients avoid skin care of any kind during this period of time, but there is the risk that patients will not comply and use their own products that may be irritating or harmful to the skin. Therefore, surgeons may want to consider providing or recommending a safe and simple regimen during this immediate phase of healing that includes a gentle cleanser and a nonactive moisturizer. A nonactive cleanser is defined as one that does not contain alpha hydroxy acids, retinols, vitamin C, or exfoliating beads. The cleanser should be one that can be easily "tissued" off instead of rinsed off. Choosing a gentle cleanser that can be "tissued" off ensures that the cleanser does not rinse back behind the ears, under the chin, or anywhere else where healing incisions may reside. The nonactive moisturizer should contain ingredients to hydrate dry, sensitive skin and gently restore the lipid barrier of the skin,

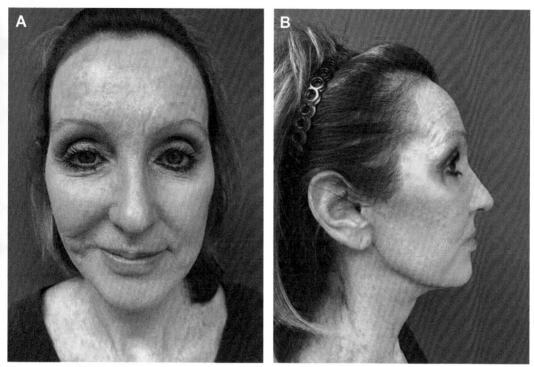

Fig. 3. Patient 1 ten months after surgery. (*A*) Anteroposterior view. (*B*) Right lateral view.

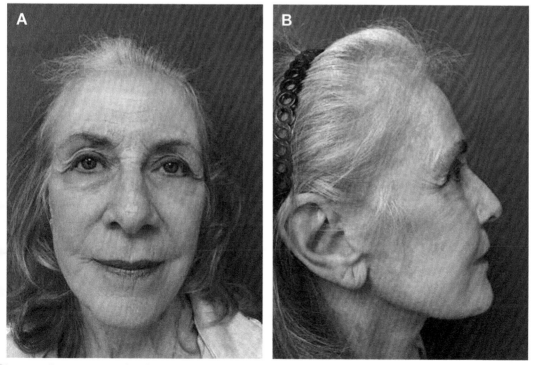

Fig. 4. Patient 2 ten months after surgery. (*A*) Anteroposterior view. (*B*) Right lateral view.

Table 2
Postoperative skincare regimen

Phase	Timing	Components and Details
Immediate	7–14 d after surgery	No topical agents OR Nonactive cleanser and moisturizer: • Nonactive cleanser that does NOT contain alpha hydroxy acids, retinols, vitamin C, or exfoliating beads • Nonactive moisturizer to hydrate dry, sensitive skin (eg, hyaluronic acid, aloe vera, ceramides, and squalene)
Interim	2–10 wk after surgery	Can begin to incorporate additional skin care products, such as antioxidants, sun protection, additional moisturizing agents. Can also apply camouflage makeup provided it is not applied over an open incision or wound
Maintenance	Beyond 10 wk after surgery	Contains similar components of preoperative skincare program

such as hyaluronic acid, aloe vera, ceramides, and squalene.

In the interim skin care phase, starting about 1 to 2 weeks after surgery to over the next 6 to 8 weeks, patients can begin to incorporate additional skin care products into their routines, like those that contain antioxidants, sun protection (mineral formulations are preferred over chemical formulations), and additional moisturizing agents, as long as the patient does not experience any irritation to those products. Camouflage or traditional makeup can be applied at that time as well, provided it is not applied over an open incision or wound. The authors' experiences demonstrate that when proper skin care is routinely applied in the immediate postoperative phase of recovery, attempts to apply makeup to conceal redness or bruising in the interim phase are more successful.

The final skin care maintenance phase has components that are similar to the components of a preoperative skin care program (if one has been prescribed) and should include the full range of products that are appropriate for each patient's skin type and specific concerns. Optimized skin health will not only complement the newly defined contours of the face that are a result of the facelift but also produce more natural-looking results because the patient's skin also has the potential to appear younger than the patient's age and to help patients "protect their investment." The time spent with patients to thoughtfully explain the postoperative phases of the skin care plan can also provide opportunities to offer additional psychosocial and emotional support and to present a more comprehensive aesthetic plan in the perioperative period.

REFERENCES

1. Khavkin J, Ellis DA. Aging skin: histology, physiology, and pathology. Facial Plast Surg Clin North Am 2011;19:229–34.
2. Janis JE. Essentials of aesthetic surgery. New York: Thieme; 2018.
3. Hubbard BA, Unger JG, Rohrich RJ. Reversal of skin aging with topical retinoids. Plast Reconstr Surg 2014;133:481e–90e.
4. Stuzin JM. MOC-PSSM CME article: face lifting Plast Reconstr Surg 2008;121:1–19.
5. Stuzin JM. Restoring facial shape in face lifting the role of skeletal support in facial analysis and midface soft-tissue repositioning. Plast Reconstr Surg 2007;119:362–76 [discussion: 377–8].
6. Mendelson B, Wong CH. Changes in the facial skeleton with aging: implications and clinical applications in facial rejuvenation. Aesthetic Plast Surg 2012;36:753–60.
7. Coleman S. Structural fat grafting. New York: Thieme Publishers; 2004.
8. Reece EM, Pessa JE, Rohrich RJ. The mandibular septum: anatomical observations of the jowls in aging-implications for facial rejuvenation. Plast Reconstr Surg 2008;121:1414–20.
9. Boros K, Freemont T. Physiology of ageing of the musculoskeletal system. Best Pract Res Clin Rheumatol 2017;31:203–17.
10. Bartlett SP, Grossman R, Whitaker LA. Age-related changes of the craniofacial skeleton: an anthropometric and histologic analysis. Plast Reconstr Surg 1992;90:592–600.
11. Hellman M. Changes in the human face brought about by development. International Journal of

Orthodontia, Oral Surgery and Radiography 1927; 13:475–516.

12. Kahn DM, Shaw RB Jr. Aging of the bony orbit: a three-dimensional computed tomographic study. Aesthet Surg J 2008;28:258–64.

13. Pessa JE, Chen Y. Curve analysis of the aging orbital aperture. Plast Reconstr Surg 2002;109:751–5 [discussion: 756–60].

14. Mendelson BC, Hartley W, Scott M, et al. Age-related changes of the orbit and midcheek and the implications for facial rejuvenation. Aesthetic Plast Surg 2007;31:419–23.

15. Rohrich RJ, Hollier LH Jr, Janis JE, et al. Rhinoplasty with advancing age. Plast Reconstr Surg 2004;114: 1936–44.

16. Pessa JE, Zadoo VP, Mutimer KL, et al. Relative maxillary retrusion as a natural consequence of aging: combining skeletal and soft-tissue changes into an integrated model of midfacial aging. Plast Reconstr Surg 1998;102:205–12.

17. Pessa JE, Peterson ML, Thompson JW, et al. Pyriform augmentation as an ancillary procedure in facial rejuvenation surgery. Plast Reconstr Surg 1999;103:683–6.

18. Pessa JE, Slice DE, Hanz KR, et al. Aging and the shape of the mandible. Plast Reconstr Surg 2008; 121:196–200.

19. Pecora NG, Baccetti T, McNamara JA Jr. The aging craniofacial complex: a longitudinal cephalometric study from late adolescence to late adulthood. Am J Orthod Dentofacial Orthop 2008;134:496–505.

20. Romo T, Yalamanchili H, Sclafani AP. Chin and pre-jowl augmentation in the management of the aging jawline. Facial Plast Surg 2005;21:38–46.

21. Little JW. Three-dimensional rejuvenation of the midface: volumetric resculpture by malar imbrication. Plast Reconstr Surg 2000;105:267–85 [discussion: 286–9].

22. Fitzgerald R, Graivier MH, Kane M, et al. Facial aesthetic analysis. Aesthet Surg J 2010;30(Suppl): 25s–7s.

23. Marten TJ. Facelift. Planning and technique. Clin Plast Surg 1997;24:269–308.

24. Nease CJ, Aldridge E, English JL. Adjunctive techniques in contemporary rhytidectomy. Atlas Oral Maxillofac Surg Clin North Am 2014;22:75–89.

25. Baker TJ. Surgical rejuvenation of the face. 2nd edition. Chicago: Mosby-Year Book; 1993.

26. Mavroforou A, Giannoukas A, Michalodimitrakis E. Medical litigation in cosmetic plastic surgery. Med Law 2004;23:479–88.

27. Lindor RA, Kunneman M, Hanzel M, et al. Liability and informed consent in the context of shared decision making. Acad Emerg Med 2016;23: 1428–33.

28. De Brauwer F, Bertolus C, Goudot P, et al. Causes for litigation and risk management in facial surgery:

a review of 136 cases. J Stomatol Oral Maxillofac Surg 2019;120(3):211–5.

29. Gogos AJ, Clark RB, Bismark MM, et al. When informed consent goes poorly: a descriptive study of medical negligence claims and patient complaints. Med J Aust 2011;195:340–4.

30. Kandinov A, Mutchnick S, Nangia V, et al. Analysis of factors associated with rhytidectomy malpractice litigation cases. JAMA Facial Plast Surg 2017;19: 255–9.

31. Spatz ES, Krumholz HM, Moulton BW. The new era of informed consent: getting to a reasonable-patient standard through shared decision making. JAMA 2016;315:2063–4.

32. Frosch DL, Kaplan RM. Shared decision making in clinical medicine: past research and future directions. Am J Prev Med 1999;17:285–94.

33. Politi MC, Han PK, Col NF. Communicating the uncertainty of harms and benefits of medical interventions. Med Decis Making 2007;27:681–95.

34. Boss EF, Mehta N, Nagarajan N, et al. Shared decision making and choice for elective surgical care: a systematic review. Otolaryngol Head Neck Surg 2016;154:405–20.

35. Ubbink DT, Santema TB, Lapid O. Shared decision-making in cosmetic medicine and aesthetic surgery. Aesthet Surg J 2016;36:Np14–9.

36. Boyll P, Kang P, Mahabir R, et al. Variables that impact medical malpractice claims involving plastic surgeons in the United States. Aesthet Surg J 2018; 38:785–92.

37. Oshima Lee E, Emanuel EJ. Shared decision making to improve care and reduce costs. N Engl J Med 2013;368:6–8.

38. Wilson SR, Strub P, Buist AS, et al. Shared treatment decision making improves adherence and outcomes in poorly controlled asthma. Am J Respir Crit Care Med 2010;181:566–77.

39. Marten E, Langevin CJ, Kaswan S, et al. The safety of rhytidectomy in the elderly. Plast Reconstr Surg 2011;127:2455–63.

40. Guyuron B, Raszewski R. Undetected diabetes and the plastic surgeon. Plast Reconstr Surg 1990;86: 471–4.

41. Baker TJSJ, Baker TM. Facial skin resurfacing. New York: Thieme Publishers; 1998.

42. Jensen JA, Goodson WH, Hopf HW, et al. Cigarette smoking decreases tissue oxygen. Arch Surg 1991; 126:1131–4.

43. Rees TD, Liverett DM, Guy CL. The effect of cigarette smoking on skin-flap survival in the face lift patient. Plast Reconstr Surg 1984;73:911–5.

44. Sorensen LT. Wound healing and infection in surgery: the pathophysiological impact of smoking, smoking cessation, and nicotine replacement therapy: a systematic review. Ann Surg 2012;255: 1069–79.

45. Barker DE. Prevention of bleeding following a rhytidectomy. Plast Reconstr Surg 1974;54:651–3.

46. Berner RE, Morain WD, Noe JM. Postoperative hypertension as an etiological factor in hematoma after rhytidectomy. Prevention with chlorpromazine. Plast Reconstr Surg 1976;57:314–9.

47. Durnig P, Jungwirth W. Low-molecular-weight heparin and postoperative bleeding in rhytidectomy. Plast Reconstr Surg 2006;118:502–7 [discussion: 508–9].

48. Grover R, Jones BM, Waterhouse N. The prevention of haematoma following rhytidectomy: a review of 1078 consecutive facelifts. Br J Plast Surg 2001; 54:481–6.

49. Jones BM, Grover R. Reducing complications in cervicofacial rhytidectomy by tumescent infiltration: a comparative trial evaluating 678 consecutive face lifts. Plast Reconstr Surg 2004;113: 398–403.

50. Jones BM, Grover R. Avoiding hematoma in cervicofacial rhytidectomy: a personal 8-year quest. Reviewing 910 patients. Plast Reconstr Surg 2004; 113:381–7 [discussion: 388–90].

51. Broughton G 2nd, Crosby MA, Coleman J, et al. Use of herbal supplements and vitamins in plastic surgery: a practical review. Plast Reconstr Surg 2007; 119:48e–66e.

52. Heller J, Gabbay JS, Ghadjar K, et al. Top-10 list of herbal and supplemental medicines used by cosmetic patients: what the plastic surgeon needs to know. Plast Reconstr Surg 2006;117:436–45 [discussion: 446–7].

53. Ramanadham SR, Costa CR, Narasimhan K, et al. Refining the anesthesia management of the facelift patient: lessons learned from 1089 consecutive face lifts. Plast Reconstr Surg 2015;135:723–30.

54. Taub PJ, Bashey S, Hausman LM. Anesthesia for cosmetic surgery. Plast Reconstr Surg 2010;125: 1e–7e.

55. Matchett RM, Carraway JH. Anesthesia and aesthetic surgery. Aesthet Surg J 1998;18:136–9.

56. Trussler AP, Hatef DA, Rohrich RJ. Management of hypertension in the facelift patient: results of a national consensus survey. Aesthet Surg J 2011;31: 493–500.

57. Baker DC, Stefani WA, Chiu ES. Reducing the incidence of hematoma requiring surgical evacuation following male rhytidectomy: a 30-year review of 985 cases. Plast Reconstr Surg 2005;116:1973–85 [discussion: 1986–7].

58. Rosso JD, Zeichner J, Alexis A, et al. Understanding the epidermal barrier in healthy and compromised skin: clinically relevant information for the dermatology practitioner: proceedings of an expert panel roundtable meeting. J Clin Aesthet Dermatol 2016; 9:S2–s8.

59. Ambro BT, Wright RJ. Depression in the cosmetic surgery patient. Facial Plast Surg 2010;26:333–8.

60. Sarcu D, Adamson P. Psychology of the facelift patient. Facial Plast Surg 2017;33:252–9.

61. Goin MK, Burgoyne RW, Goin JM, et al. A prospective psychological study of 50 female face-lift patients. Plast Reconstr Surg 1980;65: 436–42.

62. American Psychiatric Association. Diagnostic and statistical manual of mental disorders: DSM-5. 5th edition. Arlington (VA): American Psychiatric Association; 2013.

63. Greenberg JL, Weingarden H, Wilhelm S. A practical guide to managing body dysmorphic disorder in the cosmetic surgery setting. JAMA Facial Plast Surg 2019;21(3):181–2.

64. Dey JK, Ishii M, Phillis M, et al. Body dysmorphic disorder in a facial plastic and reconstructive surgery clinic: measuring prevalence, assessing comorbidities, and validating a feasible screening instrument. JAMA Facial Plast Surg 2015;17: 137–43.

65. Joseph AW, Ishii L, Joseph SS, et al. Prevalence of body dysmorphic disorder and surgeon diagnostic accuracy in facial plastic and oculoplastic surgery clinics. JAMA Facial Plast Surg 2017;19: 269–74.

66. Derby BM, Codner MA. Evidence-based medicine: face lift. Plast Reconstr Surg 2017;139: 151e–67e.

67. Maricevich MA, Adair MJ, Maricevich RL, et al. Facelift complications related to median and peak blood pressure evaluation. Aesthetic Plast Surg 2014;38:641–7.

68. Innocenti A, Ciancio F, Melita D, et al. Evidence-based medicine: face lift. Plast Reconstr Surg 2017;140(5):756–7e.

69. McKinney P, Katrana DJ. Prevention of injury to the great auricular nerve during rhytidectomy. Plast Reconstr Surg 1980;66:675–9.

70. Ozturk CN, Ozturk C, Huettner F, et al. A failsafe method to avoid injury to the great auricular nerve. Aesthet Surg J 2014;34:16–21.

71. Baker DC, Conley J. Avoiding facial nerve injuries in rhytidectomy. Anatomical variations and pitfalls. Plast Reconstr Surg 1979;64:781–95.

72. Glowacki D. Effective pain management and improvements in patients' outcomes and satisfaction. Crit Care Nurse 2015;35:33–41 [quiz: 43].

73. Bennett KG, Kelley BP, Vick AD, et al. Persistent opioid use and high-risk prescribing in body contouring patients. Plast Reconstr Surg 2019;143: 87–96.

74. Marcusa DP, Mann RA, Cron DC, et al. Prescription opioid use among opioid-naive women undergoing immediate breast reconstruction. Plast Reconstr Surg 2017;140:1081–90.

75. Brummett CM, Waljee JF, Goesling J, et al. New persistent opioid use after minor and major surgical

procedures in US adults. JAMA Surg 2017;152: e170504.

6. Sun EC, Dixit A, Humphreys K, et al. Association between concurrent use of prescription opioids and benzodiazepines and overdose: retrospective analysis. BMJ 2017;356:j760.

7. Dasgupta N, Funk MJ, Proescholdbell S, et al. Cohort study of the impact of high-dose opioid analgesics on overdose mortality. Pain Med 2016;17:85–98.

8. Aynehchi BB, Cerrati EW, Rosenberg DB. The efficacy of oral celecoxib for acute postoperative pain in face-lift surgery. JAMA Facial Plast Surg 2014; 16:306–9.

79. Berger M, Weigert R, Pascal E, et al. Assessing improvement of patient satisfaction following facelift surgery using the FACE-Q scales: a prospective and multicenter study. Aesthetic Plast Surg 2019;43(2): 370–5.

80. Litner JA, Rotenberg BW, Dennis M, et al. Impact of cosmetic facial surgery on satisfaction with appearance and quality of life. Arch Facial Plast Surg 2008; 10:79–83.

UNITED STATES POSTAL SERVICE ®

Statement of Ownership, Management, and Circulation
(All Periodicals Publications Except Requester Publications)

1. Publication Title	2. Publication Number	3. Filing Date
CLINICS IN PLASTIC SURGERY	006 – 530	9/18/2019

4. Issue Frequency	5. Number of Issues Published Annually	6. Annual Subscription Price
JAN, APR, JUL, OCT	4	$543.00

7. Complete Mailing Address of Known Office of Publication (Not printer) (Street, city, county, state, and ZIP+4®)

ELSEVIER INC.
230 Park Avenue, Suite 800
New York, NY 10169

Contact Person: STEPHEN R. BUSHING
Telephone (Include area code): 215-239-3688

8. Complete Mailing Address of Headquarters or General Business Office of Publisher (Not printer)

ELSEVIER INC.
230 Park Avenue, Suite 800
New York, NY 10169

9. Full Names and Complete Mailing Addresses of Publisher, Editor, and Managing Editor (Do not leave blank)

Publisher (Name and complete mailing address)

TAYLOR BALL, ELSEVIER INC.
1600 JOHN F KENNEDY BLVD. SUITE 1800
PHILADELPHIA, PA 19103-2899

Editor (Name and complete mailing address)

JESSICA MCCOOL, ELSEVIER INC.
1600 JOHN F KENNEDY BLVD. SUITE 1800
PHILADELPHIA, PA 19103-2899

Managing Editor (Name and complete mailing address)

PATRICK MANLEY, ELSEVIER INC.
1600 JOHN F KENNEDY BLVD. SUITE 1800
PHILADELPHIA, PA 19103-2899

10. Owner (Do not leave blank. If the publication is owned by a corporation, give the name and address of the corporation immediately followed by the names and addresses of all stockholders owning or holding 1 percent or more of the total amount of stock. If not owned by a corporation, give the names and addresses of the individual owners. If owned by a partnership or other unincorporated firm, give its name and address as well as those of each individual owner. If the publication is published by a nonprofit organization, give its name and address.)

Full Name	Complete Mailing Address
WHOLLY OWNED SUBSIDIARY OF REED/ELSEVIER, US HOLDINGS	1600 JOHN F KENNEDY BLVD. SUITE 1800 PHILADELPHIA, PA 19103-2899

11. Known Bondholders, Mortgagees, and Other Security Holders Owning or Holding 1 Percent or More of Total Amount of Bonds, Mortgages, or Other Securities. If none, check box ► ☐ None

Full Name	Complete Mailing Address
N/A	

12. Tax Status (For completion by nonprofit organizations authorized to mail at nonprofit rates) (Check one)

The purpose, function, and nonprofit status of this organization and the exempt status for federal income tax purposes:
☒ Has Not Changed During Preceding 12 Months
☐ Has Changed During Preceding 12 Months (Publisher must submit explanation of change with this statement)

PS Form 3526, July 2014 [Page 1 of 4 (see instructions page 4)] PSN: 7530-01-000-9931 PRIVACY NOTICE: See our privacy policy on www.usps.com.

---

13. Publication Title	14. Issue Date for Circulation Data Below
CLINICS IN PLASTIC SURGERY	JULY 2019

15. Extent and Nature of Circulation			Average No. Copies Each Issue During Preceding 12 Months	No. Copies of Single Issue Published Nearest to Filing Date
a. Total Number of Copies (Net press run)			269	291
b. Paid Circulation (By Mail and Outside the Mail)	(1)	Mailed Outside-County Paid Subscriptions Stated on PS Form 3541 (Include paid distribution above nominal rate, advertiser's proof copies, and exchange copies)	124	139
	(2)	Mailed In-County Paid Subscriptions Stated on PS Form 3541 (Include paid distribution above nominal rate, advertiser's proof copies, and exchange copies)	0	0
	(3)	Paid Distribution Outside the Mails Including Sales Through Dealers and Carriers, Street Vendors, Counter Sales, and Other Paid Distribution Outside USPS®	79	104
	(4)	Paid Distribution by Other Classes of Mail Through the USPS (e.g. First-Class Mail®)	0	0
c. Total Paid Distribution (Sum of 15b (1), (2), (3), and (4))			203	243
d. Free or Nominal Rate Distribution (By Mail and Outside the Mail)	(1)	Free or Nominal Rate Outside-County Copies included on PS Form 3541	50	28
	(2)	Free or Nominal Rate In-County Copies Included on PS Form 3541	0	0
	(3)	Free or Nominal Rate Copies Mailed at Other Classes Through the USPS (e.g. First-Class Mail)	0	0
	(4)	Free or Nominal Rate Distribution Outside the Mail (Carriers or other means)	0	0
e. Total Free or Nominal Rate Distribution (Sum of 15d (1), (2), (3), and (4))			50	28
f. Total Distribution (Sum of 15c and 15e)			253	271
g. Copies not Distributed (See instructions to Publishers #4 (page #3))			16	20
h. Total (Sum of 15f and g)			269	291
i. Percent Paid (15c divided by 15f times 100)			80.24%	89.67%

*If you are claiming electronic copies, go to line 16 on page 3. If you are not claiming electronic copies, skip to line 17 on page 3.

16. Electronic Copy Circulation	Average No. Copies Each Issue During Preceding 12 Months	No. Copies of Single Issue Published Nearest to Filing Date
a. Paid Electronic Copies ►		
b. Total Paid Print Copies (Line 15c) + Paid Electronic Copies (Line 16a) ►		
c. Total Print Distribution (Line 15f) + Paid Electronic Copies (Line 16a) ►		
d. Percent Paid (Both Print & Electronic Copies) (16b divided by 16c × 100) ►		

☒ I certify that 50% of all my distributed copies (electronic and print) are paid above a nominal price.

17. Publication of Statement of Ownership

☒ If the publication is a general publication, publication of this statement is required. Will be printed in the OCTOBER 2019 issue of this publication. ☐ Publication not required.

18. Signature and Title of Editor, Publisher, Business Manager, or Owner

STEPHEN R. BUSHING - INVENTORY DISTRIBUTION CONTROL MANAGER

Date: 9/18/2019

I certify that all information furnished on this form is true and complete. I understand that anyone who furnishes false or misleading information on this form or who omits material or information requested on the form may be subject to criminal sanctions (including fines and imprisonment) and/or civil sanctions (including civil penalties).

PS Form 3526, July 2014 (Page 3 of 4) PRIVACY NOTICE: See our privacy policy on www.usps.com

Moving?

Make sure your subscription moves with you!

To notify us of your new address, find your **Clinics Account Number** (located on your mailing label above your name), and contact customer service at:

Email: journalscustomerservice-usa@elsevier.com

800-654-2452 (subscribers in the U.S. & Canada)
314-447-8871 (subscribers outside of the U.S. & Canada)

Fax number: 314-447-8029

Elsevier Health Sciences Division
Subscription Customer Service
3251 Riverport Lane
Maryland Heights, MO 63043

*To ensure uninterrupted delivery of your subscription, please notify us at least 4 weeks in advance of move.

Printed and bound by CPI Group (UK) Ltd, Croydon, CR0 4YY

08/05/2025

01864746-0015